Patient Empowerment 101

More than a book, it's an adventure!

Patient Empowerment 101:

More than a book, it's an adventure!

Ann M. Hester, M.D.
Board Certified Internist

Copyright 2022 by Ann M. Hester. All rights reserved.
PatientEmpowerment101.com

Disclaimer

The information in this book is for informational and educational purposes only. It is not a substitute for your doctor's advice. This publication is designed to provide authoritative information to help you and your doctors work together more efficiently. The author accepts no responsibility for any decisions made based upon the contents of this book. All healthcare decisions should be made in consultation with your physician.

Dedication

    This book is dedicated to the Lord. Thank you for blessing me with the knowledge to help a multitude of my brothers and sisters. May everyone who is enlightened by this book look to you, the true author of wisdom. And may any praise for this work be directed solely to you. I realize that I am a mere vessel for their blessing.

Special thanks to:

- Marianne Cunanan-Bush, M.D., Internist
- Margaret E. Delgado, DNP, ACNP Board Certified
- Dr. Raymond Zarate, Doctor of Nursing Practice, Hospitalist
- Lauren Hester, BSN, RN
- M. Cornelious Musara, M.D., FACS, Surgeon
- Marc Okun, M.D., Cardiologist
- Chirag Chaudhari, M.D., Emergency Room Physician
- Tiffany Megary, M.D., Emergency Room Physician
- Sharon Nath, Emergency Room PA-C
- Victor S Dorodny, MD, ND, PHD, MPH,
   Chief Wisdom Officer @
   www.linkedin.com/in/AmazingDrD
- Dipa Mair, MSN, RN
- Erkan Hassan, Pharm.D., FCCM
- Jessica Collet Murphy, MBA, MS, RD, LD, CHC
   Healthcare Member Experience Analyst
- Dr. Tammy Porter, DNP, MLS, RN, CPHQ, CCM
- Claire Thevenot, MBA, RN, OCN, BCPA, Founder of Clarity Patient Advocates
- Anne Llewellyn, MS, BHSA, RN, CCM, CRRN, CMGT-BC, FCM Founder of NurseAdvocate.com

Table of Contents

Introduction 1

Chapter 1: See Eye to Eye With Your Doctors 5

Chapter 2: Prepare for Your Appointment 31

    Questionnaires for 11 Common Symptoms 33

Chapter 3: Choose the Doctor Right for You 57

Chapter 4: Health Insurance Options 67

Chapter 5: Your Medical Records Are Vital 85

Chapter 6: Stay Safe in The Hospital 150

Chapter 7: Technology in Health Care 177

Chapter 8: The Power of An Advocate 186

Conclusion 191

Appendix 1. Common Medical Tests 192

Appendix 2. Common Medical Abbreviations 207

Appendix 3. Glossary of Common Medical Terms 210

Introduction

Hello! My name is Ann M. Hester, M.D. and I am a board-certified internal medicine doctor. I'm not your doctor, so no need to think of me as Dr. Hester (or even Dr. Ann). I want you to think of me as your longtime friend, Ann, who just happens to be a physician. Think of this book as a conversation where I'll share words of wisdom from over 25 years of clinical experience.

Your health care is of the utmost significance. Yet, I realize that reading a book about medical issues could easily leave some snoring and others pulling their hair out with a mix of anxiety and confusion. So, I made this book unique. To make learning this material like more of a must-have adventure than a chore, there is a website. You can take quizzes, watch videos to reinforce concepts, and download charts and questionnaires found in this book. Most charts are in Word format, so you can fill them in and save them to your desktop. You can also print them and are encouraged to do so. More on that later. And don't be surprised if new information is added to the site over time. Healthcare is dynamic, and I want your experience to be as well.

Occasional levity in this book is meant to make you pause and smile. Healthcare is a serious topic and sometimes can be overwhelming. Taking a step back and looking through another lens can lessen the tension and even make you laugh a little. Some believe Bennett Cerf, a humor writer, coined the phrase, "Laughter is the best medicine." Others attribute it to a Bible Proverb, "A merry heart doeth good like a medicine: but a broken spirit drieth the bones." Whatever its origin, the saying is true. Laughter lightens the spirit and makes us feel better inside.

Get ready. This book has the potential to change your life! There are several major goals. One of the most significant is to demystify the physician-patient relationship and make the healthcare system more user-friendly, even virtually seamless. An enlightened patient can significantly optimize her own medical care whether she never finished high school or holds a Ph.D. First, she can minimize the need for redundant, painful, potentially dangerous, and often expensive tests. Next, she can help slash the time it takes her doctor to get the correct diagnosis. (So, she gets on the road to healing sooner.) She can make the healthcare system safer for her and her family as well. Yet a not-so-insignificant benefit of developing what I'll call 'patient prowess' is a tremendous potential to save money on medical bills. This book will unleash your power to take your rightful place at the center of your healthcare team. Does this pique your interest? Keep reading to begin your transformation.

America has long been facing a healthcare crisis. The loss of a job can mean the difference between having superior healthcare coverage for you and your family and having none. But millions of Americans don't benefit from employer-sponsored healthcare and struggle to receive even the most basic care. Yet no one can afford to take access to high-quality healthcare for granted. No one knows what tomorrow will bring.

According to data published by the Association of American Medical Colleges (AAMC), America could face a shortage of between 54,100 and 139,000 physicians by the year 2033. Sadly, this alarming number does not even reflect the high number of people with barriers to healthcare access, such as those who live in rural areas and some minorities. If underserved Americans used the healthcare system like the majority of citizens, the demand could increase by an additional 74,100 to 145,500 physicians.

Another significant finding is the projected growth of the population aged 65 and over is about 45.1% by 2033, compared to an overall population growth rate of 10.4% during the same period. Naturally, an office visit for a 70-year-old with several chronic medical problems will be more time intensive than one for a healthy 40-year-old, but we all want and deserve access to an attentive physician. We all want to know our physician will have time to see us whenever we become ill.

Imagine a shortage of thousands of physicians in your state in the not-so-distant future. What will healthcare be like? How long will you have to wait to see a primary care physician? What about a specialist?

The mere thought is enough to bring on goosebumps. While the future of healthcare is uncertain, there are things everyone can do to improve his outlook. Learning how to communicate with medical professionals and expedite your diagnosis can go a long way in optimizing your health care future. So, how will this book help you weather the storm? I'm so glad you asked.

This book will teach you:
- How to help expedite your diagnoses for the rest of your life
- What your doctor will want to know about your illness
- How to get the most out of every doctor's visit
- Why advance preparation can help slash your medical bills
- The importance of developing a personal copy of your medical records
- Essential things to take with you to the doctor's office
- Tips for selecting the doctor right for you
- Basics of different types of health insurance
- How to optimize your safety whenever you are hospitalized
- How to use technology to improve your health care
- Why you need an advocate for your healthcare
- Common medical tests and terms
- Frequently used medical abbreviations
- A glossary of commonly used medical terms, along with a pronunciation key
- Words of encouragement and inspiration from multiple different professionals in the medical field
- And more!

We are all keenly aware that, in some ways, the practice of medicine is moving from being a compassionate profession to a robotic system. Doctors are frustrated. Patients are frustrated. At times, this "new and improved" healthcare system seems like it churns patients in and out of a revolving door. Insurance companies must contain costs, just like every other type of business. Otherwise, they would go bankrupt, just like every other type of business. There must be a healthy balance between providing excellent care and managing the costs of that care. If several major health insurance companies folded, imagine how many people would abruptly find themselves without acceptable healthcare coverage. Fortunately, national guidelines based on sound medical research help guide healthcare decisions. Still, cost-containment is a necessity for America's healthcare system to thrive and provide excellent care. It's important to remember that.

Meanwhile, numerous doctors are fed up with the changes in the system. Many are paid significantly less for their services than in the past. Even worse, less of their typical day is devoted to direct patient care because of all the bureaucratic and administrative demands they face. For a variety of reasons, many doctors are leaving the field sooner than they once thought.

No one knows where this merry-go-round will take us as a society. Concerns over access to care, potential rationing of care, and no care have many Americans sitting on the edge of their seats. Yet, you can play a proactive role. You may not have a medical background. You may not have a personal advocate in Congress, but you can become the best advocate possible for your own health care. The better informed you are, the more you can help your physicians help you. You'll find the URLs for the webpages to reinforce your knowledge on the last page. Now, let's get started!

Chapter 1

SEE EYE TO EYE WITH YOUR DOCTORS

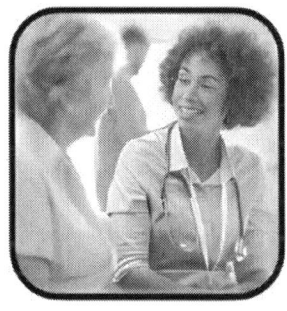

Becoming a knowledgeable patient can dramatically change your health care trajectory. A lasting result of learning how to navigate the healthcare system is that you will help minimize healthcare expenditures and decrease medical waste. This is good for your wallet and for the strength of our healthcare system. But, again, this is an added benefit, not the primary goal.

While physicians and other healthcare providers devote many years to studying medicine, patients simply don't have a comparable patient school to attend to learn how to navigate the healthcare system. This book helps fill that void by teaching you how to think more like doctors and nurses. You won't be able to hold a high-level conversation with a neurosurgeon simply by reading this book. But you can make healthcare professionals stand up and notice they are dealing with a well-informed patient. With the right tools you can play a significant role in expediting and optimizing your own healthcare. This will push your interactions with medical personnel to a much higher level, a definite win-win situation. Once you develop a stronger sense of what is important to them and what is not, you and your healthcare providers can walk side by side in your journey to optimize your health and the care you receive.

Most patients do not understand how to communicate effectively and efficiently with their healthcare providers. Think about it. The layperson cannot be expected to grasp intricate physiologic and anatomic principles it took their physicians many years to learn. And truth be told, doctors often forget that medical terminology is not second nature to that precious person seated in front of them on the examining room table. Unfortunately, this disparity is often the basis for missed or delayed diagnoses, excessive testing, and inadequate treatment.

> *Optimal patient outcomes can be achieved via patient-provider partnerships delivering appropriate, accessible, affordable care when and where it's needed.*
>
> **-Victor S. Dorodny, MD, ND, PHD, MPH, Chief Wisdom Officer @www.linkedin.com/in/AmazingDrD**

The result is that the patient-physician relationship is frequently not as harmonious as it could or should be. A patient does not come into the office and say, "Doctor, I've been searching the internet, and I am sure I have an overactive thyroid. After extensive online research, I've decided I want to be treated with radioactive iodine. Now, all I need for you to do is order the test to confirm my suspicion." Whew! If it were really that simple, MD really would stand for Mountain Doctor (as Granny Clampett in the old sitcom The Beverly Hillbillies claimed). And her grandson Jethro Bodine really could be a brain surgeon with a 6th-grade education.

Physicians are trained to listen to the "presenting complaints" of patients. Then they work backward by asking them questions, performing a physical examination, and finally devising a mental list of possible diagnoses *(list of differential diagnoses)* that could account for their symptoms.

After obtaining this preliminary information, they focus on ordering tests to "rule in or rule out" specific diagnoses that seem most likely. The stronger the suspicion is about a particular illness the fewer tests are needed to confirm that diagnosis. So, if your history is communicated clearly, there is tremendous potential to save significant money and time. But, more important, you will be treated promptly and efficiently with the least amount of risk and discomfort from what could prove to be unnecessary testing.

Potential results of poor doctor-patient communication

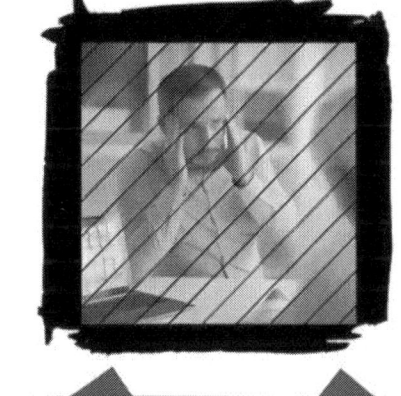

- excessive testing
- multiple procedures
- missed diagnosis
- ineffective medication
- extra follow-up visits
- too much time off work
- high medical bills
- poor outcomes
- prolonged suffering

The thrust of this chapter is to give you an overview of how to communicate with your physicians to accomplish these goals. This is no easy task. Patients tell their stories in a manner natural for them. We all do. At the same time, physicians concentrate on pulling out the pertinent facts and discarding the rest.

Naturally, it is advantageous to understand some of the key points your doctor will want to know about your current illness before you even step into your doctor's office. Typically, patients mentally pull together their recollection of their sickness while sitting on the examining table, sometimes assisted by a family member. But what if you're in pain? What if you are wearing a paper robe as you sit on a cold table? Or, what if you simply don't recall the answers to his questions?

This approach is time-consuming. It is also frustrating for you and, yes, even for your physician. Taking this approach may lead you to forget to mention very important nuances of your illness, especially if you are already nervous or uncomfortable. Meanwhile, your doctor may feel overwhelmed with the 12 sick patients left to be seen in the next 3 hours and try to cut to the chase of your problem. In this common scenario, you may feel rushed, intimidated, or devalued.

Naturally, this would only escalate any baseline anxiety and fear. This is not a win-win situation for anyone. But, if you have thought through your problem beforehand and you're prepared to tell a brief yet information-packed short story about your illness by the time your doctor steps foot in your room, you will have overcome an enormous hurdle most patients never do. Patients were never taught how to speak the language their doctors speak. How would you know what the doctor is looking for if no one ever explained this to you?

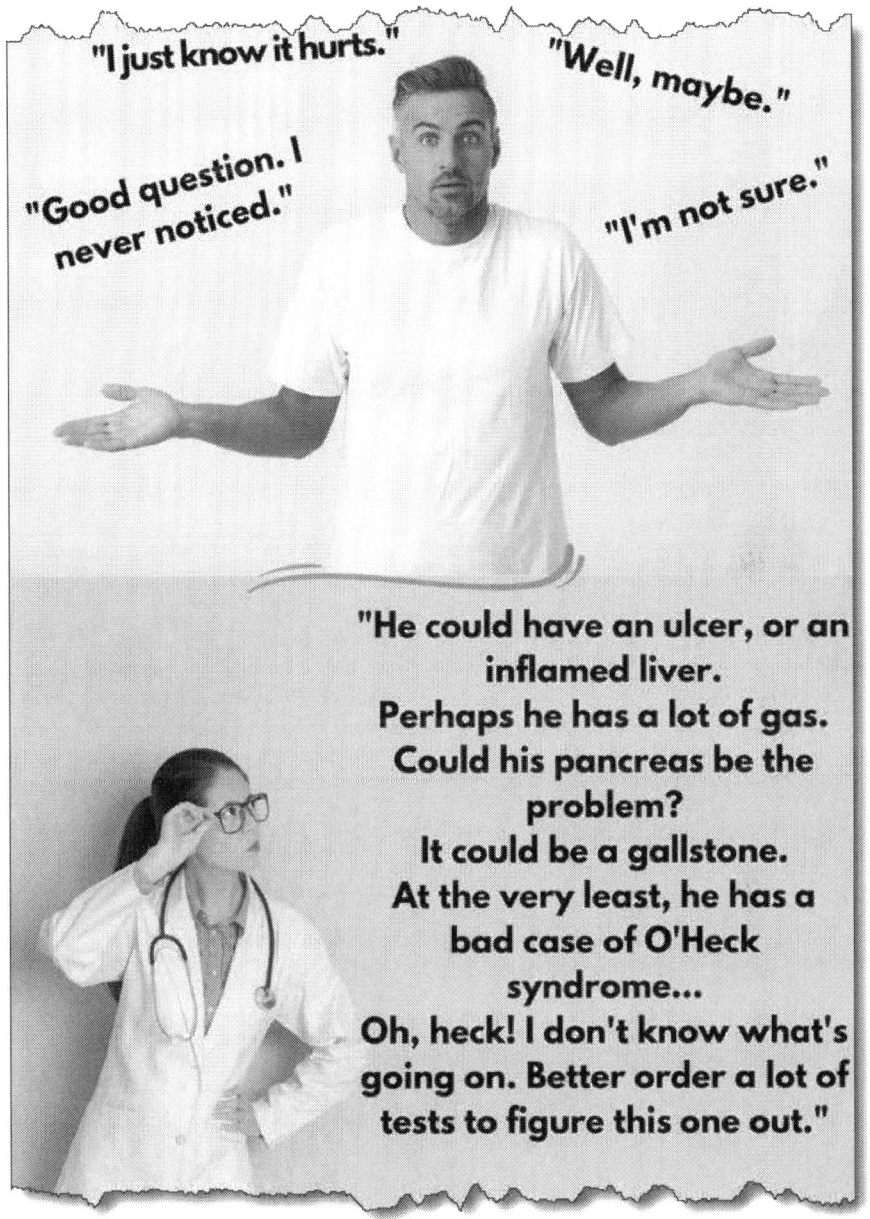

So, let's talk about what will help your doctor help you quickly and efficiently. There are eight vital elements surrounding your sickness. Doctors call this your *History of Present Illness (HPI)*. In simpler terms, there are eight essential things your doctor may ask about your current illness. These factors are part of national *Evaluation and Management (E/M)* guidelines. Insurance company reimbursements to doctors are directly linked to E/M guidelines. Doctors cannot routinely charge for the highest possible level of reimbursement. Instead, they must 'earn it'. Here, earning it means documenting an appropriate level of detail for each medical visit.

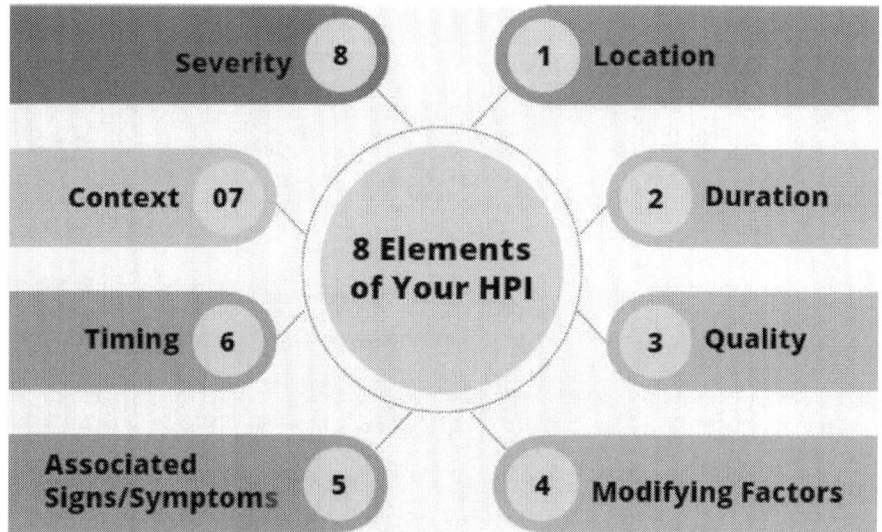

Elements of Your HPI (history of present illness)

Remembering this list of eight elements can be challenging. Developing a memory aid to help you remember them is worthwhile. Here is an example:

A **QUALITY** action movie needs a great **LOCATION**. The **TIMING** of the star's first entrance should be based on the **ASSOCIATED CONTEXT** of what is going on now. The director should **MODIFY** the **DURATION** of each scene based on the **SEVERITY** of the situation.

Quality

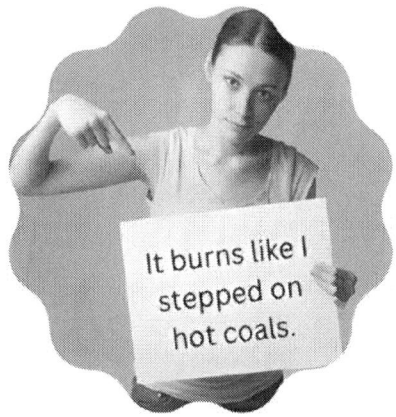

It burns like I stepped on hot coals.

Location

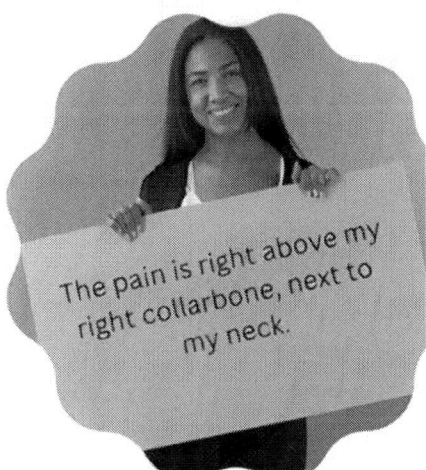

The pain is right above my right collarbone, next to my neck.

Timing

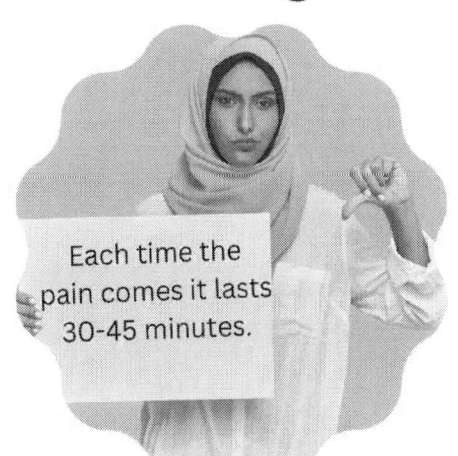

Each time the pain comes it lasts 30-45 minutes.

Associated Signs/Symptoms

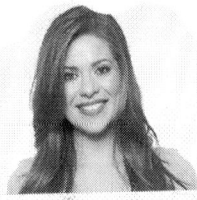

When my stomach hurts, I feel like I want to vomit.

Context

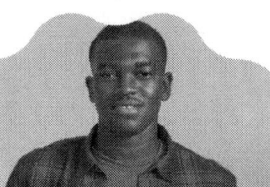

My back pain started immediately after I tripped over my wife's new shoes and landed on my tailbone.

Modifying Factor

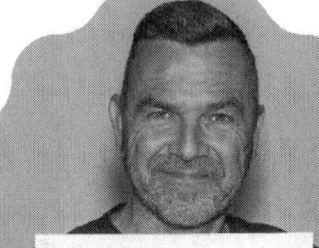

A full-strength aspirin makes my headache go away within 30 minutes.

Duration

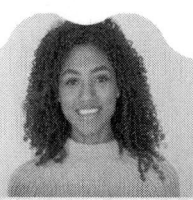

My symptoms have been constant for three days.

Severity

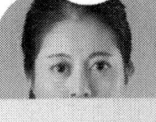

My back pain is so bad it's very hard to get out of bed each morning. I can barely walk.

Hint: Doctors may ask you to rate your pain on a scale of 1-10.

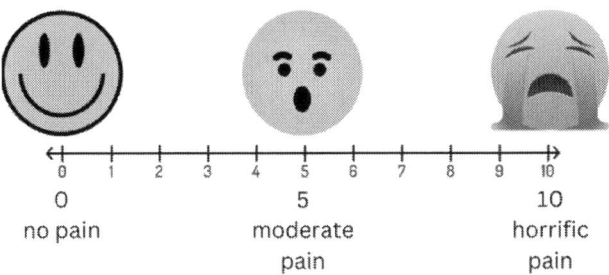

Doctors must be able to prove the amount they charged the insurance company for your visit is in line with these national Evaluation and Management (E/M) guidelines. Otherwise, they risk fines, big ones, should they be audited. They could even be charged with healthcare fraud and face a prison term! So, it's easy to see why physicians must meticulously document in your medical record.

But it's not all about the money by any means. These eight designated elements are instrumental in helping a physician understand what the diagnosis is and what it is not. For instance, if you tell your doctor 3 days ago (**timing**) you developed mild (**severity**), sharp (**quality**) pain in the upper left abdomen (**location**) immediately after lifting heavy weights (**context**), and the pain gets worse whenever you twist your upper body (**modifying factors**), you can rest assured, you doctor is not going to order expensive tests looking for evidence of appendicitis. Your appendix is in your lower right abdomen, and nothing you said would make a doctor focus on an inflamed appendix as your diagnosis. Instead, she'll probably do a quick examination and treat you for a muscle strain. All eight elements may not be needed for every illness, but it is good to consider each one.

Let's take a deeper dive into how giving details can expedite your (correct) diagnosis. This example is simply meant for illustrative purposes. Later on, you will be given a chart with details of signs and symptoms to look for if you develop abdominal pain. You can even download this list and make copies for every time you experience pain in the abdomen.

Ready? So, let's say a person has abdominal pain, her doctor will want to know several key features to help pin down the diagnosis. When the abdominal pain is in the upper right abdomen, doctors think about the organs that lie in that area, such as the liver, gallbladder, stomach, or pancreas. Other conditions can cause pain in the upper right abdomen, even skin conditions. Still, when a patient complains of pain in that region, anatomically speaking, doctors must strongly consider conditions like hepatitis, gallstones, gastritis (stomach inflammation), an ulcer, or inflammation of the pancreas. Other diseases, such as appendicitis, are possible but less likely.

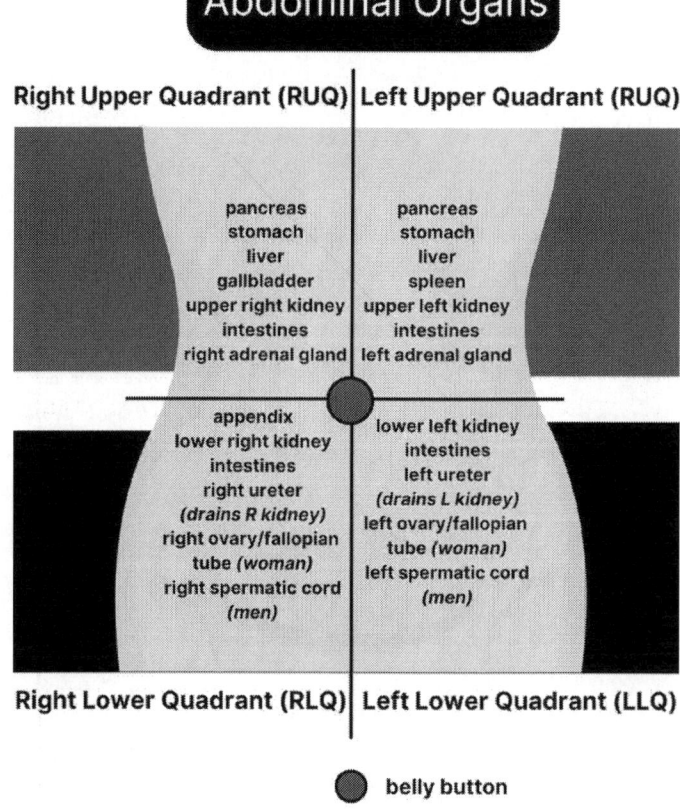

Also, suppose fevers and chills accompany the abdominal pain. There, the reason for the pain is more likely to be related to infection than if they do not. And, if over-the-counter antacids help the pain, it is more likely due to an acid-related condition, such as an ulcer or gastritis. This therapy should not significantly affect other causes of pain.

Radiation of pain is also essential to consider. If upper abdominal pain radiates straight through to the back, pancreatitis and an ulcer are high on the list of possibilities. Gallbladder disease is highly likely if it radiates to the right shoulder blade.

Then the character comes in. **Hint:** This is not meant to conjure up thoughts about the chill-creating scene of your favorite movie when the underdog steps in to save the day. This character has to do with the details of the pain. For instance, is the pain a burning sensation, as sometimes occurs with indigestion? Is it a dull, achy type of pain? Is it crampy?

Your physician may also want to know if this is the first time this specific type of pain has occurred. If not, did you seek medical attention in the past, and if so, were any tests done to evaluate the pain? For example, let's say you had similar pain in the upper right abdomen intermittently for several months, and your previous physician ordered an abdominal ultrasound. This test showed no gallstones, so your new doctor will focus her attention on other potential causes of your pain.

If you are not sure of the names of the tests done in the past and their results, precious time could be wasted trying to obtain your old records. Or the doctor may simply repeat a slew of expensive tests so she can get answers fast. So, it may come down to your money or your safety. Guess which will take precedence? The result is that it costs more money to obtain the diagnosis, and the diagnosis may be significantly delayed.

It is also important to acknowledge other symptoms associated with the pain, though they may be less troublesome. For example, let's say a person has also been coughing up yellow sputum (mucus/phlegm mixed with saliva). The cause of the upper abdominal pain may be pneumonia in the lower right lung and not a disease in the abdominal cavity itself. But if this person has recently noticed that his stools are black and sticky, he may have internal bleeding due to an ulcer.

The chronological sequence of the pain is also significant. For instance, if abdominal pain has been present and gradually increasing over several days, it could be due to hepatitis, gastritis, or ulcers, to name a few things. It is less likely to be due to a slow-growing tumor which takes months to significantly enlarge.

Many illnesses cause vomiting, but the timing of the vomiting and its character are also important. If a person occasionally vomits a couple of hours after eating, the doctor may consider different diseases than if he consistently vomits immediately after eating.

The appearance of the vomitus matters as well. For example, suppose Sue has a stomach virus which causes her to wretch and vomit. Frequent vomiting may cause excessive stress on the esophagus which may cause a blood vessel to rupture. This can cause Sue to vomit bright red blood.

This is a different scenario from John with a bleeding ulcer as a cause of vomiting blood. Blood can irritate the lining of his stomach and induce vomiting. The first time he throws up he may vomit bright blood if the bleeding is brisk. Alternatively, he may have a slow leaky bloody vessel and throw up "coffee grounds" or dark, gritty-looking vomitus. This is because blood mixed with the acid in the stomach turns brown and gritty. John may have bloody or coffee ground vomitus from the beginning. In Sue's case the vomitus consisting of food and clear fluid eventually turned bloody when the situation became more prolonged and complicated, resulting in trauma to a blood vessel.

Delving further into the issue of vomiting, your doctor may want to know if you vomit up everything you eat and drink or if the vomiting is occasional and not associated with eating. If it is associated with eating, how much time passes after eating before you vomit? How many times a day do you vomit? A little vomitus twice a week, provided there is no evidence of blood, usually will not do much harm if you stay hydrated. However, if you have been vomiting several times a day, you may be at risk of becoming dehydrated. You also risk having a potentially severe alteration in the concentration of vital components of the blood, such as a low potassium level. Here, you may need hospitalization and intravenous fluids until you can obtain regular nourishment.

Besides vomiting, other vital issues need to be addressed. Is there diarrhea or constipation? If there is diarrhea, how many stools are you having a day? Are the stools loose, well-formed, or watery? Do you have to get up during the night to go to the bathroom? Can you hold your bowel movements until you reach the commode? Is there blood or mucus in the stools? Is each bowel movement a large or small amount? Suppose you are having many large-volume watery bowel movements a day. There, you may also be at risk for dehydration and changes in the chemical composition of the blood.

How many stools have you had in the past week if you are having constipation? How does that compare to your norm? Constipation could be due to inadequate fiber in the diet, a thyroid disorder, medications that cause constipation, diabetes mellitus, or a host of other diseases. Still, frequently it is due to no identifiable illness.

A simple complaint such as abdominal pain can have a multitude of different causes. For instance, a person may see her doctor because her stomach has been aching for a few weeks. She may not have thought her constipation was significant because she has gotten used to it. However, after talking to the patient and examining her, the doctor may feel it is worthwhile to assess her thyroid gland. Upon doing so, he finds that her thyroid gland is underactive, causing her to be constipated. Constipation turns out to cause her abdominal pain. The solution is to treat her thyroid disorder, which may be the sole cause of constipation and the root of her stomach pain.

Many potential diagnoses could cause abdominal pain, including:
- ulcers
- pancreatitis (pancreas inflammation)
- gastritis (stomach inflammation)
- hepatitis (liver inflammation)
- gallstones/gallbladder inflammation

- appendicitis (appendix inflammation)
- pneumonia
- irritable bowel syndrome
- constipation
- diabetes mellitus
- psychological issues
- gastroenteritis ('stomach flu')
- and many more!

It could be time-consuming and expensive to reach a diagnosis for a complaint as basic as abdominal pain. The preceding is only a partial list. However, with a good history and physical examination, physicians usually need few tests to confirm their suspicion of a diagnosis.

That is where you can play a tremendous role in helping your doctor help you. An excellent historical account of the illness from the patient is often the most important factor in making the correct diagnosis, really!

When a medical school professor told the class I didn't believe him. How could a patient's words be as vital in helping a doctor make the correct diagnosis as the advanced medical technology I read so much about? But it didn't take long to make me a believer. Some conditions are best diagnosed with blood tests or imaging, such as X-rays, CAT scans or MRIs. But think back. How often have you gone to see your doctor and left without an order for any tests? Common things are common, and when a doctor has seen or read about a condition repeatedly making that diagnosis can be a piece of cake.

Next, let's look at another example. This compares two qualities of historical accounts by a patient.

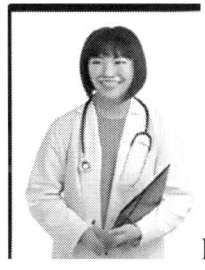 **Dr. Chen:** "Hello, Mr. Jones. What brings you to the office today?"

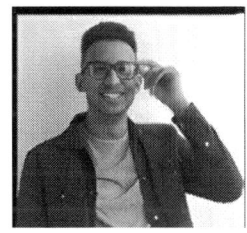 **Mr. Jones:** "Doc, I've been having a burning sensation in the middle of my upper abdomen for several months now. I was sitting in front of the television the first time I noticed it, not doing anything unusual. It's not always there, but when it starts, it's severe. It lasts several minutes to a few hours at a time and then goes away, but it comes back, maybe a few days or weeks later. Sometimes it even wakes me up in the middle of the night. I can't pinpoint what brings it on, but when I have the pain, it gets better a few hours after I eat some- thing. The pain does not move anyplace, my appetite has been good, and I have had a little nausea but no vomiting. My bowel habits haven't changed. I still have one well-formed stool every day. I haven't tried any medication for the pain since I know food usually helps. I'm not having any other problems, and other than this annoying stomach pain, I feel great. My mother and brother also have similar stomach problems. What do you think is wrong with me?"

This patient has practically given his doctor his diagnosis. His symptoms are most concerning for an ulcer. In less than a minute, he gave a concise, detailed explanation of his presenting complaint. You can do the same using the symptoms forms provided in this book.

He told his doctor:
- What he was doing the first time he noticed the pain (was watching television)
- When he first noticed the pain (several months ago)
- The character of the pain (burning)

- And the severity of the pain (fairly severe as opposed to mild and almost negligible)
- The location of the pain (mid-upper abdomen)
- The radiation of the pain (none)
- How long the pain lasts when it comes (minutes to hours)
- And what things seem to bring on the pain (no identifiable causes)
- What relieves the pain (food)
- How long it takes for relief to occur (a few hours)
- How effectively food relieves the pain (it sometimes returns)
- Other symptoms or lack thereof
- Other symptoms specifically related to his gastrointestinal tract (nausea, no vomiting, regular bowel movements)
- Other symptoms, or lack thereof, related to other systems of his body ("Other than this annoying stomach pain, I feel great.")
- Others close to him with similar symptoms (two close relatives)

(Don't worry about the details this early. We will delve into all this and more later.)

This patient has provided such a good history that his doctor would have a good idea of how she plans to treat him by the time he finishes his last sentence.

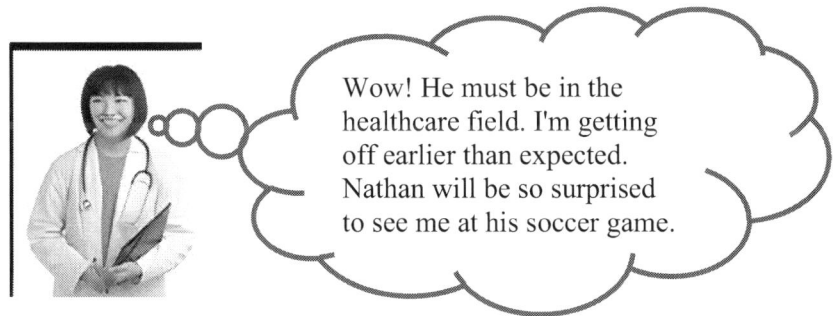

Wow! He must be in the healthcare field. I'm getting off earlier than expected. Nathan will be so surprised to see me at his soccer game.

There would be no need to order an expensive (potentially painful) battery of tests to get to this diagnosis because the doctor was given such an excellent history. By the end of this book, YOU will be that type of patient. Stay tuned.

After a targeted physical examination, she may give him a trial of antiulcer medication and see him back soon to see how well it worked. She may order one or two focused diagnostic tests.

Compare this previous example to:

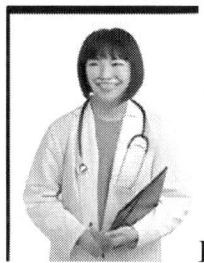

Dr. Chen: "Hello, Mr. Jones. What can I do for you today?"

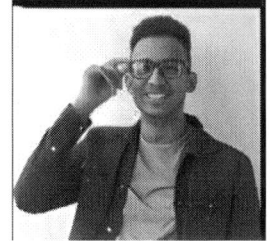

Mr. Jones: "My stomach hurts."
Dr. Chen: "How long has it been a problem?"
Mr. Jones: "Doc, I have been having stomach pain for a long time."

There is a pause. The doctor is thinking, 'A long time means different things to different people. One person means several years, while another means several days.'

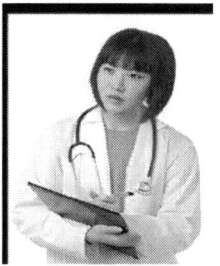

Dr. Chen: "Sir, what do you mean by a long time? Do you mean it has been hurting for a matter of days, weeks, months, or years?"

Mr. Jones: "I'm not sure when it first started. I just know it has been going on a long time."

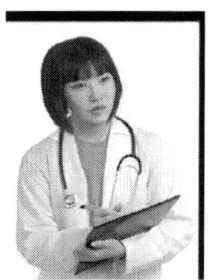

The doctor is thinking, 'Okay, I need to help him pin down a general time frame for his symptoms.'
Dr. Chen: "Did you first notice this pain before or after January of this year?"
Mr. Jones: (Pause to reflect.) "It must have been before because Uncle Lorenzo and Aunt Joi came to visit for Christmas, and I remember that I ate something over the holiday that made me feel terrible. I almost called in to work sick, but I decided to go on in any way."

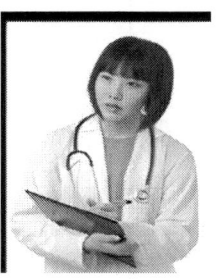

The doctor is thinking, 'Well, I know his abdominal pain must have been going on at least five months since this is May.'

Dr. Chen: "Where does it hurt?"
Mr. Jones: "Most of the time, it hurts under my rib cage on the right side."
Dr. Chen: "Most of the time? Where else does it hurt?"
Mr. Jones: "I don't pay it any attention. It just seems to hurt all over."

Dr. Chen: "Well, take a moment and give it some thought."
Mr. Jones: (Pause.) "Sometimes it moves to the middle."
Dr. Chen: "Does the pain ever go thru to your back?"
Mr. Jones: "Sometimes."
Dr. Chen: "Is your pain constant, or does it come and go?"
Mr. Jones: "Well, it's not always there. It just hurts sometimes."
Dr. Chen: "How often do you have this pain?"
Mr. Jones: "Oh, I guess a few days a month."
Dr. Chen: "Is the pain constant for those days, or does it wax and wane?"
Mr. Jones: "It waxes and wanes, I guess."
Dr. Chen: "How long does it last when it comes?"
Mr. Jones: "It usually lasts a few hours, but sometimes it hurts all day and all night."
Dr. Chen: "Is it worse when it begins or when time wears on?"
Mr. Jones: "I think when it begins."
Dr. Chen: "Is the onset gradual or abrupt?"
Mr. Jones: "I guess it comes on pretty fast."
Dr. Chen: "When you have this pain, does anything make it better or worse?"
Mr. Jones: "Not that I can think of."
Dr. Chen: "Have you tried any over-the-counter medication?"
Mr. Jones: "Not really. Well, I'm not sure."
Dr. Chen: "Does food make the pain better or worse?"
Mr. Jones: "You know, I never paid any attention to how food affects it, if at all. Wait! I take that back. Once I ate a huge beef taco and that made me feel awful. But, uh, on second thought, it just gave me a lot of gas. When I passed the gas, I felt better."
Dr. Chen: "What does the pain feel like? For instance, is the pain sharp, dull, or crampy?"
Mr. Jones: "All I know is that it hurts like, like wow!

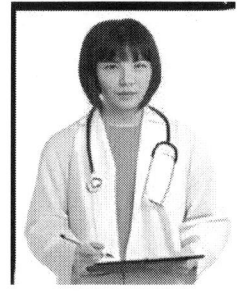

The doctor is thinking, 'I really need to know the character of this pain. Let me try something else.'

Dr. Chen: "Would you characterize the pain as an ache, a stabbing pain as if someone were sticking a fork in your belly, like a grabbing and letting go sensation, or ..."

Mr. Jones: "It's an aching sensation, probably."

Dr. Chen: "When you have this pain, do you have any other accompanying symptoms, such as nausea and vomiting?"

Mr. Jones: "Sometimes I feel like I want to throw up, but I don't."

Dr. Chen: "Have your bowel movements changed in any manner?"

Mr. Jones: "I get constipated sometimes."

Dr. Chen: "How long do you go without having a bowel movement?"

Mr. Jones: "Most of my life, I have had a bowel movement every day, but every now and then, I miss a day. But last week, my wife made some killer pinto beans, and I ate a ton. You can imagine how that went (chuckle)."

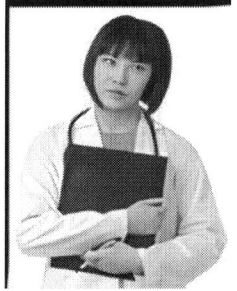

The doctor is thinking, 'This is not true constipation.'

Dr. Chen: "Have you noticed anything about your bowel habits since you started having this abdominal pain? For instance, has the color or consistency of the stool changed, or have you noticed any blood or mucus in your stool?

Mr. Jones: "Well, recently, I have had dark stools, but I thought that was due to eating kale."

Dr. Chen: "Are they black and tarry or just darker than usual?"

Mr. Jones: "Doc, I really don't pay that much attention to my bowel movements. That's kinda disgusting, don't you think? I can't even stand changing my son's diaper. I'm certainly not going to examine my own stools. Makes me sick on my stomach just to think about it. Yuk!"

Dr. Chen: "Has anything else been bothering you?"

Mr. Jones: "Sometimes my right shoulder aches."

Dr. Chen: "Does this coincide with your stomach pain?"

Mr. Jones: "I never noticed."

Dr. Chen: "Which did you notice first, the abdominal pain or the shoulder pain?"

Mr. Jones: "I really couldn't tell you."

Dr. Chen: "Do you have any fevers or chills?"

Mr. Jones: "Sometimes I get a little warm."

Dr. Chen: "Have you taken your temperature recently?"

Mr. Jones: "No."

This conversation could go on and on and on because the list of potential causes of this patient's abdominal pain is extensive. Yet, there are still additional questions to ask before developing the mental list of differential diagnoses. The doctor probably may order more tests than if she had a clear picture of what was happening. It is unrealistic to expect the layperson to understand what is essential and what is not. That will come with time and practice.

Likewise, you cannot be expected to communicate a perfect history to your healthcare providers unless you have been trained in the medical field, but reading this book is a huge step in the right direction. Still, there are basic questions you should run through your mind before you see your doctor. Doing so can dramatically expedite your communication and your diagnosis.

When relaying an explanation about an illness, these things should be considered:

1. When did you first notice the symptoms? You don't have to pinpoint the exact time but try to recall how long ago you first noted the problem, such as two days ago, two weeks ago, or two months ago.
2. Has anyone around you, or related to you, had similar problems? Some conditions are contagious, while others commonly run in families.
3. Describe the chronological sequence of the symptoms.
    example: "At first, I noticed the pain every day, but over the past month it has been coming less and less frequently. Now, I only notice it once or twice a week."
4. Describe the severity of the symptoms or relate them to their impact on everyday activities.
    example: "My symptoms have been mild, and I can work and do my regular activities without difficulty."
5. If the symptom is pain, does it move anyplace, or does it remain in one place?
6. Describe the quality of the pain. Physicians commonly use terms like dull, sharp, piercing, achy, throbbing, burning, or tight to describe pain. Describe the symptom.
    example: "It feels like someone is punching me in my stomach."
7. Are the symptoms constant, or do they come and go?
8. Is the intensity the same or does it wax and wane?
    example: "I feel short of breath all the time, but it seems to be worse by the end of the day."
9. If they are intermittent, how long do the symptoms last each time they are noted, and how long of a reprieve do you have between attacks?

> *example:* "When I have chest pain, it lasts for 15 to 20 minutes at a time and then goes away for a few days before it comes back."

10. What other symptoms, if any, accompany the problem?
    > *example:* "I have noticed when I have chest pain, I often break out in a sweat and feel nauseated."
11. What things improve or worsen the symptom?
    > *example:* "Aspirin improves my headaches."
12. Do the symptoms improve on their own, or should you take something for relief? How long does it take to notice this improvement if something brings comfort?
    > *example:* "I have noticed that the pain goes away on its own within a few minutes of its inception."
13. Have you ever been evaluated by a physician for this problem in the past? If so,
    - What tests were done? (be specific)
    - What diagnosis was given?
    - What treatment was prescribed?
    - Did that treatment help?
    - Why did you stop seeing that doctor?

Please note not all questions are pertinent to all patients' symptoms. During any medical encounter, you will not be asked all the preceding questions about any given complaint. You may be asked additional questions not listed here as well. Still, take the time to think about the questions listed above. Also, common symptoms, such as abdominal pain and back pain, have downloadable, fillable charts to help you chart important details. Over time, you will learn much about what is and is not significant to your physician.

Remember different doctors have different styles. Your doctor may ask you to relate your symptoms, at which time you can give a concise history of your present illness. But she may take charge of the encounter and ask targeted questions. Regardless of the style of your personal physician consider the questions above before going to the doctor's office. Then you will be prepared to promptly answer questions, which frees up more time in the visit to potentially address other issues. You can help your doctor help you more efficiently if you think through important issues in the doctor's diagnostic decision-making process. If there are any associated symptoms not listed in the charts provided write them down.

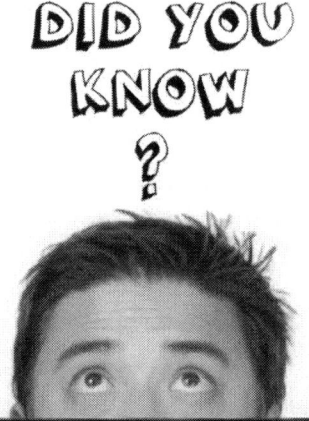

After your doctor talks to you, examines you, and reviews your test results, she will determine her "Assessment and Plan" for that visit. This is her impression about what is going on with you and what she plans to do about it, such as order a test or write a prescription. At the end of each visit, whether in the office or hospital, ask your doctor her Assessment and Plan for the day. If she looks surprised and asks if you are in the medical field, just smile and softly chuckle under your voice.

It is essential to realize that time is money. Patient encounters are "coded" for the level of care commensurate with the time spent and the complexity of the diagnosis. Poor historical information, extensive questioning, a more detailed examination, and numerous laboratory tests can be costly for you, even if your diagnosis is basic. However, suppose you could describe your symptoms, and the doctor only needs three additional minutes to do a focused exam. There, you stand to save a lot of money and get a correct diagnosis on the first visit.

Despite being concise in relating details of your illness it is crucial to be thorough. Do not be consumed by the clock on the wall or feel like you are a failure if your doctor needs to spend considerable time with you. The most important thing is your health. It is unrealistic to believe that you will become an expert at being a patient by reading this or any book. Even physicians are not expert patients when they become ill. [We're known to be pretty bad patients, but that's another story.] Do your best to help your doctor help you. Your input will be appreciated. Always remember an accurate medical history can be lifesaving in certain situations. You are the *first* line of defense against your own illnesses and must be well-informed!

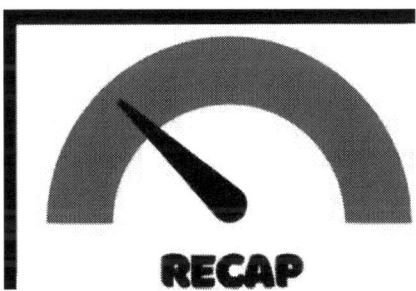

- Develop a memory aid to help you remember the eight elements of your history of present illness (HPI).
- Prepare for a visit to the doctor when you first feel ill.
- The doctor's Assessment and Plan is her impression of the cause of your symptoms and what she plans to do next.
- Take your time and relay your symptoms to your doctor in a concise, methodical manner.

QUIZ

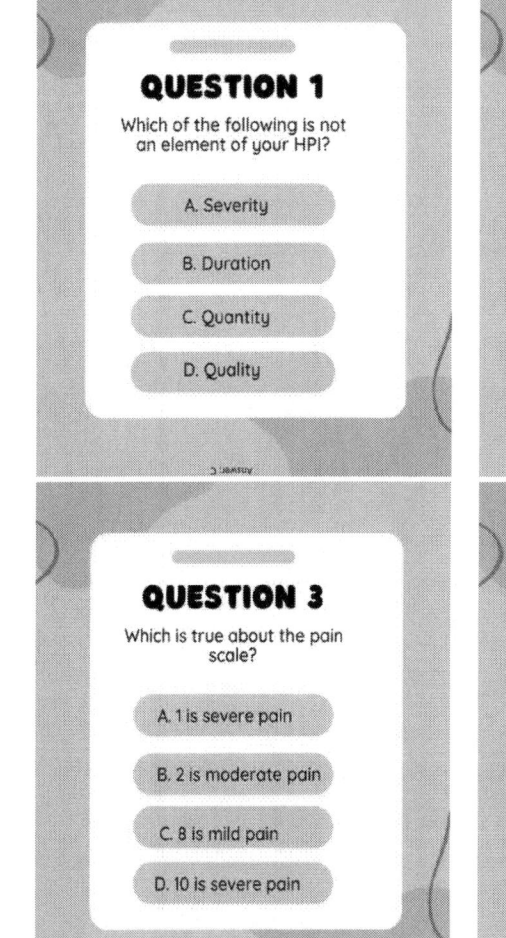

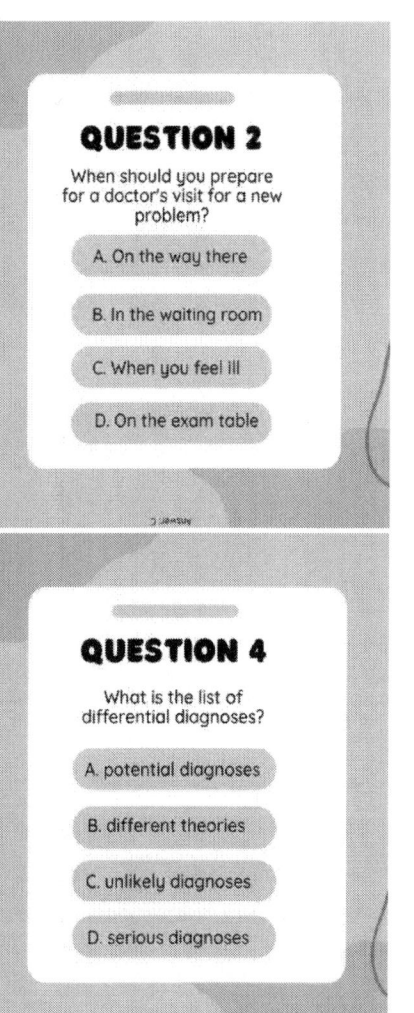

QUESTION 1
Which of the following is not an element of your HPI?

A. Severity

B. Duration

C. Quantity

D. Quality

QUESTION 2
When should you prepare for a doctor's visit for a new problem?

A. On the way there

B. In the waiting room

C. When you feel ill

D. On the exam table

QUESTION 3
Which is true about the pain scale?

A. 1 is severe pain

B. 2 is moderate pain

C. 8 is mild pain

D. 10 is severe pain

QUESTION 4
What is the list of differential diagnoses?

A. potential diagnoses

B. different theories

C. unlikely diagnoses

D. serious diagnoses

Chapter 2

PREPARE FOR YOUR APPOINTMENT

So, you've made an appointment to see your doctor. Now what? Prepare for the visit in advance. By now, you have a good idea of the questions your doctor will ask you for a new problem, such as a new cough or abdominal pain. But how do you prepare for a routine follow up visit for a chronic problem, such as high blood pressure?
Regardless of the visit type, take the following:

- Insurance card
- Your medications/medication list
- List of your questions for the day. Prioritize the questions in order of their importance to you. If you run out of time, you want to make sure the most pressing issues were addressed and not pushed back to a future appointment.
- Any pertinent outside documents germane to the visit
- Your personal health records (if this is your first visit).

In a later chapter you will learn how to develop a concise, organized copy of these records. If, instead, you bring in a copy of every medical visit, diagnosis, test result, and hospitalization for the past 30 years, beware...

What you may see.

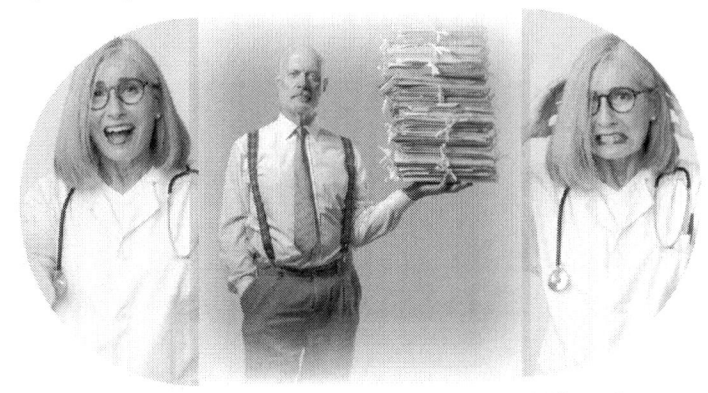

What she may feel.

If you are going in for a follow-up visit for a chronic problem, be prepared with pertinent information your doctor may want. For instance, if you have asthma, she may ask how well your asthma has been controlled since your last visit. If you have high blood pressure, bring in a log of your blood pressure readings, preferably taken at different times of the day. Likewise, if you have diabetes, your blood sugar log would be most appreciated.

> ❝ You must be an active participant with your health. Research (credible sources) and ASK questions. We have more control over our lives than we think. Yes, some things in health and in life will happen to us without explanation, but it's the steps you take after that are in your control.
> **-Lauren Hester BSN, RN** ❞

If you are seeing a doctor for an acute medical issue, remember to think thru the eight elements of the HPI discussed in chapter one. Below you will find charts to address specific questions pertaining to common medical problems. This is not an exhaustive list. But it includes some of the most common symptoms that lead people to seek medical attention. Print a copy of these charts for quick access should you become sick.

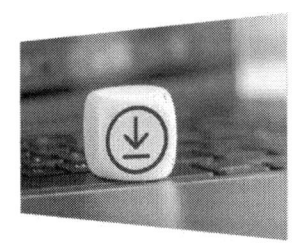

http://www.patientempowerment101.com/symptoms

Put them in a side pocket of your personal medical records binder or keep a separate folder for the blank copies. Also, save a copy to your desktop. You can even print them. They are in Word format, so you can fill in the forms by clicking boxes and typing your answers in the blank boxes. Study the forms before you go to the doctor so you can quickly answer some of the most asked questions about your symptoms. You can also take the form with you if you think you may forget something important.

SYMPTOMS

- Abdominal pain
- Chest pain
- Cough
- Diarrhea
- Fever
- Headache
- Joint pain
- Low back pain
- Rash
- Upper respiratory infection
- Shortness of breath

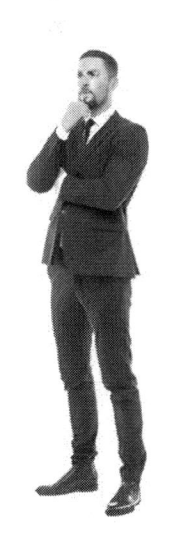

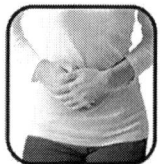

abdominal pain

1. Which part of your abdomen hurts?	Right upper quadrant ☐	Left upper quadrant ☐	Epigastric ☐	
	Right lower quadrant ☐	Left lower quadrant ☐	Umbilical ☐	
	Pelvic ☐			
2. Does the pain radiate anywhere?	Yes ☐ No ☐	If so, where?		
3. Have you had nausea or vomiting?	Yes ☐ No ☐			
4. What were you doing when you first noticed the pain?				
5. What does the vomitus look like?				
6. How long have you had this pain?				
7. On a scale of 1 to 10, how bad is the pain? (1 = mild, 10 = excruciating)	1 ☐ 2 ☐ 3 ☐ 4 ☐ 5 ☐	6 ☐ 7 ☐ 8 ☐ 9 ☐ 10 ☐		
8. What makes the pain worse?				
9. What makes it better?				
10. Do you have diarrhea currently?	Yes ☐ No ☐			
11. Describe the diarrhea.	Soft ☐ Loose ☐ Watery ☐	Small amount ☐ Medium amount ☐ Large amount ☐		
12. Is the pain at its worst when it begins or as time goes by?				

13.	How many episodes of diarrhea do you have each day?	Less than 3 ☐ 3-6 ☐ 6-9 ☐	Over 9 ☐
14.	Do you feel constipated?	Yes ☐ No ☐	If yes, explain:
15.	How long does each episode of pain last?		
16.	How does food affect the pain, if at all?		
17.	How is your appetite?		
18.	Have you had fevers or chills?		
19.	Has your abdomen been distended/bloated?		
20.	Have you had excessive belching or flatulence (passing gas from the rectum)?	Yes ☐ No ☐	If yes, explain:
21.	Have you had similar symptoms before?	Yes ☐ No ☐	If yes, explain:
22.	Have you noticed any black, tarry stools?	Yes ☐ No ☐	If yes, explain:
23.	If you have noticed blood, describe.	On tissue only ☐ Mixed with stool ☐ Blood with no stool ☐	
24.	Have you experienced any changes in your urinary habits or pain when you urinate?	Yes ☐ No ☐	If yes, explain:
25.	Do you take over-the-counter pain medications, such as aspirin or ibuprofen, on a regular basis?	Yes ☐ No ☐	If yes, explain:
26.	Has there been a recent change in your diet?	Yes ☐ No ☐	If yes, explain:
27.	Have you traveled recently?	Yes ☐ No ☐	If yes, explain:

28. Have you had any abdominal surgeries?	Yes ☐ No ☐	If yes, explain:
29. If so, did you have a laparoscopic procedure?	Yes ☐ No ☐	If yes, explain:
Women only:		
30. When was your last menstrual period?		
31. Are your menstrual cycles regular?	Yes ☐ No ☐	
32. Have you had abnormal discharge?	Yes ☐ No ☐	If yes, explain:
33. Do you have fibroids?	Yes ☐ No ☐	
34. Do you have endometriosis?	Yes ☐ No ☐	

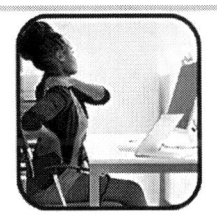

back pain

1.	What were you doing when your first noticed the pain? (e.g., playing basketball, sitting down)	
2.	Is the pain constant, or does it come and go?	Constant ☐ Intermittent ☐
3.	What effect has it had on your everyday activities? (e.g., unable to work, no effect)	
4.	Does the pain radiate anyplace, such as down your leg?	Yes ☐ If yes, explain: No ☐
5.	What makes the pain better and what makes it worse? (e.g., twisting makes it worse)	
6.	Have you had any change in your bowel or bladder habits? (e.g., urinating more frequently, difficulty initiating or stopping urine or bowel movements)	
7.	Was the onset gradual or abrupt?	Gradual ☐ Abrupt ☐
8.	Have you experienced a fever or chills?	Yes ☐ If yes, explain: No ☐
9.	Have you recently had any trauma to your back, such as with lifting heavy furniture?	Yes ☐ If yes, explain: No ☐
10.	Have you experienced any weakness or abnormal sensations in your arms or legs?	Yes ☐ If yes, explain: No ☐
11.	How do the following maneuvers affect the pain: walking, standing, bending, sitting, lying?	Walking: Standing: Bending: Sitting: Lying:

12. What is the exact location of the pain?	
13. Does your urine smell particularly foul?	Yes ☐ No ☐
14. Do you feel a burning sensation when you urinate?	Yes ☐ No ☐

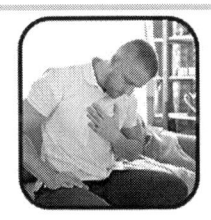

chest pain

Call 911 for concerning chest pain.

1.	How often do you have the pain?	
2.	Does the pain radiate anyplace, such as the shoulders, neck, or jaw?	Yes ☐ If so, where? No ☐
3.	What things bring on the pain and what things make it go away? (e.g., exertion brings it on and it goes away within one to two minutes of resting)	
4.	What position is the most comfortable for you when you are experiencing the pain?	
5.	Have any of your close blood relatives had a heart attack, and if so, who were they and what were their ages when they had their first attack?	Yes ☐ No ☐
6.	Do you (or did you) smoke?	Yes ☐ No ☐
7.	Have you ever been told you have a high cholesterol level?	Yes ☐ No ☐
8.	Does taking a deep breath or coughing affect the pain?	Yes ☐ No ☐
9.	Does pressing on your chest reproduce the same type of pain?	Yes ☐ No ☐
10.	Describe the pain character, i.e., pressure or squeezing sensation, sharp, achy, burning, or dull	
11.	Have you been belching or passing gas more than usual?	Yes ☐ No ☐
12.	What have you tried for the pain? Did it work, and if so, how long did it take to help?	

13. Is the pain its worst at its onset or as time moves on?		
14. Have you been diagnosed with asthma?	Yes ☐	
	No ☐	
15. Have you had trauma to your chest?	Yes ☐	
	No ☐	
16. Have you noted an unusual rash on your chest?	Yes ☐	
	No ☐	
17. Did you first notice the pain when you were physically active or were you at rest?		
18. Can you pinpoint the area of pain with a finger or is the pain the more diffuse?		
19. Does it hurt to swallow?	Yes ☐	
	No ☐	
20. Have you noticed pain or swelling in a leg?	Yes ☐	
	No ☐	
21. Is any medication/drug associated with bouts of chest pain?	Yes ☐	
	No ☐	
22. Have any of the following symptoms accompanied the chest pain?		
o Shortness of breath	Yes ☐	No ☐
o Sweating	Yes ☐	No ☐
o Nausea	Yes ☐	No ☐
o Vomit	Yes ☐	No ☐
o Lightheadedness	Yes ☐	No ☐
o Weakness	Yes ☐	No ☐
o Indigestion	Yes ☐	No ☐
o Fatigue	Yes ☐	No ☐
o Heart racing	Yes ☐	No ☐
o Radiation of the pain	Yes ☐	No ☐
23. Have you had breast pain? (women)	Yes ☐	
	No ☐	

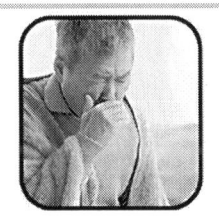

cough

1.	Do you now/did you ever smoke cigarettes?	Yes ☐ If yes, explain: No ☐
2.	Does your cough occur mainly during the daytime, nighttime, while at work, or at any time?	
3.	How long ago did you first notice the cough?	
4.	Do you ever cough after eating?	Yes ☐ No ☐
5.	Does your chest hurt when you cough?	Yes ☐ No ☐
6.	Do you sweat a lot at night (to the point of drenching your clothes)?	Yes ☐ If yes, how long? No ☐
7.	Is there a time of day when your cough is worse than at other times?	Yes ☐ If yes, explain: No ☐
8.	What is the quality? (high-pitched or low-pitched cough)	High-pitched ☐ Low-pitched ☐
9.	How intense is the cough? (mild, incapacitating, etc.)	
10.	Is the cough dry or does it produce sputum (phlegm)?	Dry ☐ Wet ☐ If wet, describe:
11.	Is the cough seasonal?	Yes ☐ No ☐
12.	Are there smokers in your house?	Yes ☐ No ☐
13.	Have you ever had pneumonia or asthma?	Yes ☐ If yes, explain: No ☐

14. Have you had a fever?	Yes ☐ No ☐	If yes, explain:
15. Are there any new odors in the house? (e.g., new paint, sprays)	Yes ☐ No ☐	
16. Do you have chest pain when you cough?	Yes ☐ No ☐	
17. Have you had shortness of breath?	Yes ☐ No ☐	
18. How frequent is the cough? (a few times a day, hourly, etc.)		
19. Does wheezing sometimes accompany the cough?	Yes ☐ No ☐	
20. Have you noticed any leg swelling recently?	Yes ☐ No ☐	
21. What things can you associate with an improvement or worsening of the cough? (e.g., exposure to dust at work worsens the cough and the cough completely subsides on weekends)		
22. Have you noticed any postnasal drip or need to clear your throat regularly?	Yes ☐ No ☐	
23. How does lying down affect the cough?		
24. Have you recently been exposed to anyone with a respiratory infection?	Yes ☐ No ☐	If yes, explain:
25. How frequently do you cough?		
26. Have you had any recent medication changes?		

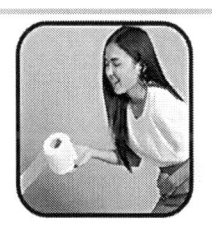

diarrhea

1.	Have you noticed any blood or mucus in the diarrhea?	Yes ☐ No ☐	
2.	Have you had fevers or chills?	Yes ☐ No ☐	If so, how high?
3.	Have you taken antibiotics in the past 45 days?	Yes ☐ No ☐	
4.	Does the diarrhea wake you up at night?	Yes ☐ No ☐	
5.	Have you been in the hospital or nursing home recently?	Yes ☐ No ☐	
6.	Have you eaten any food recently that tasted old?	Yes ☐ No ☐	
7.	How many stools have you had a day, on average?		
8.	Have your stools been black?	Yes ☐ No ☐	
9.	Are the stools of normal, low, or high volume? (normal amount, small amount, or large amount compared to a normal bowel movement?)		
10.	Describe your stools > well-formed, soft, loose, greasy, or watery.		
11.	Have you had abdominal pain, nausea, or vomiting?	Yes ☐ No ☐	If yes, describe:
12.	If you have abdominal pain, does having a bowel movement affect the pain?	Yes ☐ No ☐	If yes, describe:

13. What over-the-counter medications have you tried for the diarrhea, if any?		
14. Has anyone with whom you've been in close contact had similar symptoms?	Yes ☐ No ☐	
15. Have you traveled recently?	Yes ☐ when: No ☐	If so, where and
16. Do you drink water from the municipal water supply?	Yes ☐ No ☐	
17. Have you had any recent exposures to animals?	Yes ☐ No ☐	
18. What is the color of your stools and how does this compare to your normal stools?		
19. Have you recently taken a laxative for constipation?	Yes ☐ No ☐	
20. Have you started any new medications lately?	Yes ☐ No ☐	
21. Do you have a weakened immune system?	Yes ☐ No ☐	

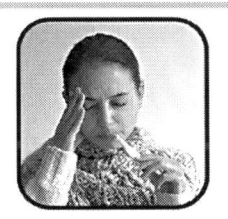

fever

1.	Have you checked your temperature, and if so, what was the highest reading?	Yes ☐ No ☐	If yes, explain:
2.	How long have you had the fever?		
3.	Do you do outdoors activities, such as hiking?	Yes ☐ No ☐	If yes, explain:
4.	Do over-the-counter medications break the fever, and if so, for how long?	Yes ☐ No ☐	If yes, explain:
5.	Which medications have you tried?		
6.	Have you recently traveled, and if so, where?	Yes ☐ No ☐	If yes, where?
7.	Have you had any recent exposures to animals?	Yes ☐ No ☐	If yes, explain:
8.	Have you recently had an animal or insect bite?	Yes ☐ No ☐	If yes, explain:
9.	Has anyone around you recently experienced a fever?	Yes ☐ No ☐	If yes, explain:
10.	What is the fever pattern? (e.g., intermittent)		
11.	Have you felt confused with the fever?	Yes ☐ No ☐	If yes, explain:
12.	Have you lost weight unexpectedly?	Yes ☐ No ☐	If yes, explain:
13.	Do you have chills?	Yes ☐ No ☐	If yes, explain:
14.	Do you have intense sweating with the fevers?	Yes ☐ No ☐	
15.	Have you recently started taking a new medication?	Yes ☐ No ☐	If yes, explain:

16. Have you had any of the following symptoms?
    - Headaches or neck stiffness
    - Light or sound sensitivity
    - Sore throat, ear or sinus pain
    - Runny nose or sneezing
    - Chest pain
    - Cough or shortness of breath
    - Abdominal pain
    - Nausea, vomiting or diarrhea
    - Decreased appetite
    - Burning when you urinate
    - Bloody or foul-smelling urine
    - Need to urinate more than usual
    - Urgency to urinate
    - Back or bone pain
    - Muscle or joint aches/swelling
    - Fatigue
    - Rash
    - Leg swelling/tenderness/redness
    - Unusual redness, heat, or tenderness of an area of skin/ new wounds
    - Vaginal discharge (women)
    - Penile discharge or testicular pain (men)

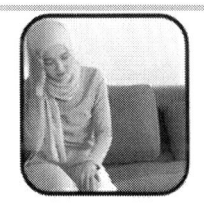

heaache

1.	Do you have a personal or family history of migraines?	Yes ☐ No ☐
2.	What is the location of the headache? (e.g., forehead, around right temple)	
3.	Is the headache throbbing, aching, tight, sharp, or dull?	
4.	What time of the day are the headaches their worst?	
5.	Do the headaches wake you up at night?	Yes ☐ No ☐
6.	Do you experience nausea or vomiting with the headaches?	Yes ☐ If yes, explain: No ☐
7.	Do you experience fevers with the headaches?	Yes ☐ No ☐
8.	Is your neck stiff?	Yes ☐ No ☐
9.	Have you had any recent tooth problems?	Yes ☐ No ☐
10.	Do any foods or beverages bring on the headaches?	Yes ☐ If yes, explain: No ☐
11.	Do menstrual cycles seem to bring on the headaches? (women only)	Yes ☐ No ☐
12.	How long do the headaches last each time? (minutes, seconds, hours, days, weeks)	
13.	What do you do to relieve the headaches? (e.g., lie down, take acetaminophen or aspirin)	

14. Have you recently started any new medications?	Yes ☐ No ☐	If yes, explain:
15. Do you take medication daily, or almost daily to relieve your headaches?	Yes ☐ No ☐	If yes, explain:
16. Do you experience any sensitivity to light, eye pain, or jaw weakness with the headaches?	Yes ☐ No ☐	If yes, explain:
17. Was the onset gradual or abrupt?		
18. Is this the worst headache of your life?	Yes ☐ No ☐	
19. Do you experience any abnormal sensations, such as strange smells, before the headaches?	Yes ☐ No ☐	If yes, explain:
20. Have you recently noticed any nasal discharge?	Yes ☐ No ☐	If yes, explain:
21. Is the headache on both sides of the head or only on one side (which side)?		
22. How does coughing or straining affect the headache?		
23. Have you had any strange sensations or weakness in your extremities?	Yes ☐ No ☐	If yes, explain:
24. How many caffeinated beverages do you drink each day? (e.g., two 8-oz cups of coffee)		
25. Does stress on the job or in the home bring on your headaches?	Yes ☐ No ☐	
26. Do you seem to make more tears than usual during headaches?	Yes ☐ No ☐	

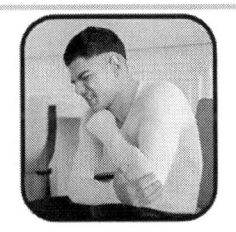

joint pain

1.	Which joints are involved?	
2.	Has there been any heat, swelling, redness, or tenderness	Yes ☐ If yes, explain: No ☐
3.	Was there any trauma to the joint, and if so, what was the mechanism of injury? (e.g., twisting, blunt trauma, a fall	
4.	Is there a family history of joint diseases?	Yes ☐ If yes, explain: No ☐
5.	What medications have you tried to alleviate the pain?	
6.	Has a fever accompanied the joint pain?	Yes ☐ If yes, explain: No ☐
7.	Do you have morning stiffness?	Yes ☐ If yes, explain: No ☐
8.	How does physical activity impact the pain?	Yes ☐ If yes, explain: No ☐
9.	Have you been engaging in more strenuous activity than usual recently?	Yes ☐ If yes, explain: No ☐

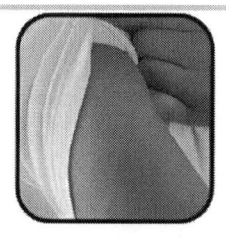

rash

1. Describe the appearance of the rash in detail. Use terms such as:
    o blisters
    o localized
    o diffuse
    o flat or raised
    o size of the average patch
    o hives
    o color of rash	

2. Describe the location of the rash.	
3. Describe the progression of the rash, such as "It began on my hands and legs and within two days also moved to my chest and back."	
4. Does the rash itch or hurt?	Yes ☐ No ☐
5. Does the rash burn?	Yes ☐ No ☐
6. How extensive was the rash at its peak? (e.g., involved one hand, entire body)	
7. Has there been a fever? (how high?)	Yes ☐ No ☐
8. Has there been any recent contact with plants or other substances?	Yes ☐ No ☐
9. Have you recently been exposed to ticks or other insects?	Yes ☐ If yes, explain: No ☐
10. Are you up to date on all the immunizations your doctor recommended?	Yes ☐ No ☐

11. Have you had measles, rubella, or chickenpox in the past?	Yes ☐ No ☐	If yes, explain:
12. Did you start a new medication recently?	Yes ☐ No ☐	If yes, explain:
13. What medications have you tried for the rash?		
14. Is this the first time experiencing a rash of this sort?	Yes ☐ No ☐	If no, explain:
15. Is the rash constant, or does it come and go?		

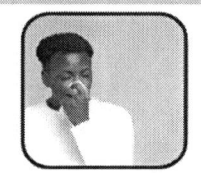

respiratory infection

1.	Do you have any nasal discharge?	Yes ☐ If yes, explain: No ☐
2.	Have you been coughing?	Yes ☐ No ☐
3.	If you have noticed a cough, is your cough dry or does it produce sputum? (What color is the sputum?)	
4.	How long have your symptoms lasted thus far?	
5.	Have you had a fever or chills?	Yes ☐ No ☐
6.	Have you noticed sneezing, a sore throat, red eyes, nausea, vomiting, or appetite change?	Yes ☐ If yes, explain: No ☐
7.	What over-the-counter medications have you tried?	
8.	Does anyone in your household smoke cigarettes?	Yes ☐ No ☐
9.	Do you have a sore throat?	Yes ☐ No ☐
10.	Has anyone around you had a respiratory infection recently?	Yes ☐ No ☐
11.	Have you been exposed to Covid-19?	Yes ☐ No ☐
12.	Have you noticed any swollen lymph glands in your neck?	Yes ☐ No ☐
13.	Have your tonsils been red, swollen, or covered with pus?	Yes ☐ No ☐

14. Has your appetite changed?	Yes ☐ No ☐	If yes, explain:
15. Have you had any nausea or vomiting?	Yes ☐ No ☐	
16. How long has your throat been sore?		
17. Does it hurt to swallow?	Yes ☐ No ☐	

shortness of breath

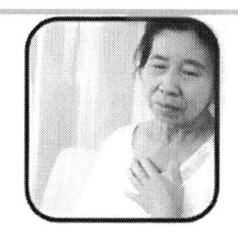

1.	How long have you felt short of breath?	
2.	Are you short of breath all the time or only during certain times of the day, or after certain activities?	
3.	How much activity does it take to make you feel short of breath? (i.e., walking 2 miles vs walking up a flight of stairs)	
4.	Do you have a history of asthma or other respiratory illnesses?	Yes ☐ If yes, explain: No ☐
5.	Have you, or has anyone around you heard wheezing sounds?	Yes ☐ No ☐
6.	Do your lips or fingers ever look bluish?	Yes ☐ If yes, explain: No ☐
7.	Do you ever wake up during the night gasping for breath?	Yes ☐ If yes, explain: No ☐
8.	How many pillows do you sleep on?	
9.	Do you get short of breath when you exert yourself?	Yes ☐ If yes, explain: No ☐
10.	Do you (or did you ever) smoke tobacco?	Yes ☐ If yes, explain: No ☐
11.	How much does shortness of breath limit your daily activities, if at all?	
12.	Have you been coughing?	Yes ☐ If yes, explain: No ☐
13.	Have you noticed leg swelling?	Yes ☐ If yes, explain: No ☐

14. Have you been coughing lately?	Yes ☐ No ☐	If yes, explain:
15. Do you have chest discomfort when you feel short of breath?	Yes ☐ No ☐	If yes, explain:
16. Have you lost weight unexpectedly recently?	Yes ☐ No ☐	If yes, explain:
17. What things make your shortness of breath better or worse? (e.g., shortness of breath improves when you sit still)	Yes ☐ No ☐	If yes, explain:
18. Do you notice excessive sweating when you feel short of breath?	Yes ☐ No ☐	
19. Does anxiety seem to precede or follow the shortness of breath?	Yes ☐ No ☐	If yes, explain:

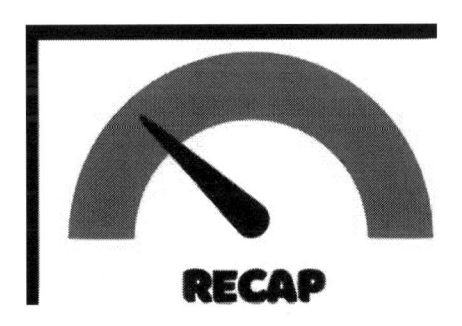

RECAP

- Remember to prepare for each visit to the doctor.
- Make use of the symptom charts provided.
- Prioritize your list of concerns.
- Be concise and precise.
- Know your medications.

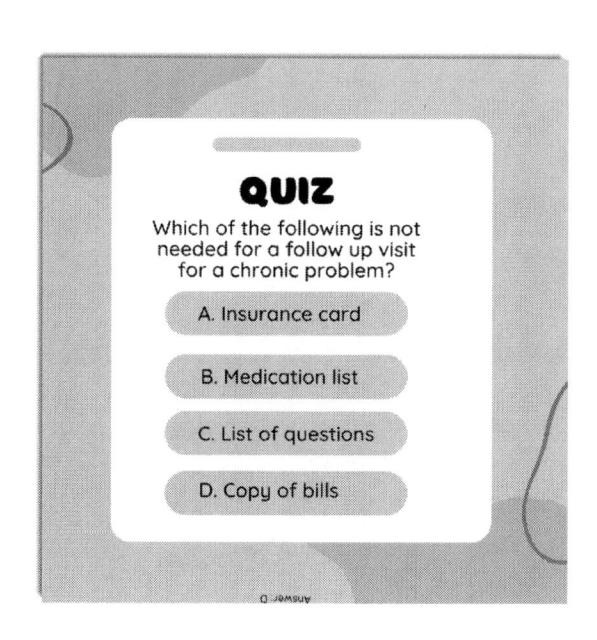

QUIZ

Which of the following is not needed for a follow up visit for a chronic problem?

A. Insurance card

B. Medication list

C. List of questions

D. Copy of bills

Answer: D

Chapter 3

CHOOSE THE DOCTOR RIGHT FOR YOU

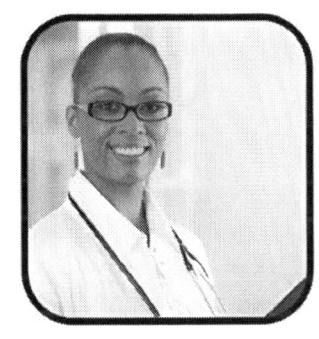

Selecting the right primary care physician can be a daunting task. You want to find a compassionate doctor. She should be attentive to your needs and concerns. And she should be highly competent. Where do you begin? Below are suggestions to streamline this process for primary care doctors and for specialists. Please take all the time you need to find the doctor whom you feel you can work with to address your healthcare needs. Don't shy away from asking questions. Remember, you want a doctor who will respect your feelings and beliefs, even if they differ from their own. Mutual respect is vital in this, and every important relationship.

Check your insurance company's provider list

If your health insurance plan requires you to see one of the providers on its panel, start there. You will find a list of contracted providers on its website or an explanation of how to obtain a list. Some companies provide this in writing to their customers. When you select a doctor, call the office and make sure the doctor still accepts your insurance. The website might need updating.

You don't want to invest a lot of time researching a physician who isn't in your plan. You can pay for visits out of pocket if you so desire. But why waste money if you can find excellent doctors in your plan? Since that can be costly, unless there is a compelling reason you want to see a specific doctor, start with your insurance company's provider panel.

If you have a specific hospital you prefer, ask if the doctor has privileges there. Although these days, many primary care physicians opt not to go to the hospital. Instead, their patients are admitted to hospital specialists, called ***hospitalists***.

Ask for recommendations

Learning about the experiences others have had with a doctor you are considering seeing is invaluable. This is often a good indicator of what you can expect should you choose this physician. But don't get so caught up in others' recommendations you overlook important details. The perfect doctor for your sister may not be the perfect one for you. Do your due diligence. You are looking for the individual you will entrust your health to. Your ideal doctor is one you can work comfortably with to reach the mutual goal of optimizing your health.

Look for board certification

Board certification requires passing a rigorous board exam and participating in ongoing medical education. Check if your potential doctor is board certified. The American Board of Medical Specialties is an excellent place to start. https://www.abms.org/verify-certification. However, not all providers are included on this website. You can visit your state medical board's website to obtain this information as well.

Investigate malpractice and medical board discipline history

The next step is to research the doctor's malpractice history. But remember, even excellent doctors make mistakes. They are as human as you. Don't automatically rule out a doctor who has been practicing for decades and has 1 or 2 malpractice claims. But if there are excessive claims, beware. Also, check to see if he has ever been disciplined by the state medical board.

Research the doctor online

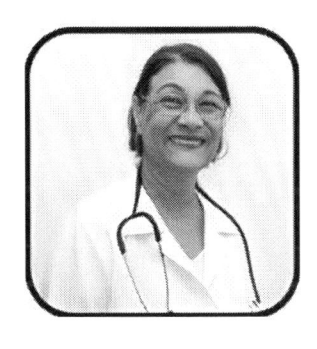

There are many websites for researching doctors. One of the most robust websites is **Care Compare**, a site of the Centers for Medicare and Medicaid Services, also known as CMS. You can find doctors and other clinicians based on location and specialty. Even if you don't have Medicare or Medicaid, this is a site to become familiar with. It provides valuable information about a variety of providers and facilities, including:

- Doctors/clinicians
- Hospitals
- Dialysis facilities
- Nursing homes and rehab services
- Inpatient rehabilitation services
- Long-term care hospitals
- Home health services
- Hospice care

Eight original **Provider Compare** websites were combined into one. On this site, you can find virtually any provider you need. In addition, you can compare providers and facilities in your area and much more. To navigate this site, start at the homepage for Care Compare listed below. Fill in your address and keywords. Choose the provider type you are interested in, and you will be presented with a wealth of useful information to help you make important decisions about your health care.

Remember that some providers' profiles may not be on this website. But as a single source, Care Compare is extremely useful for various reasons. You can find much information on current and future medical providers and facilities on one site. Providers and facilities are given star ratings on a variety of quality measures. Remember inclusion on this site is not an endorsement.

In addition, you can weigh in on the quality of your healthcare as well. You have the right to file a complaint against a doctor, provider, or facility. Examples include unsafe conditions such as fire safety concerns in a nursing home. Sloppy housekeeping at a hospital is another example. To file a complaint about a provider, visit your state's medical board for information on how to do so. If you have a complaint against a hospital, contact your state's department of health services.

Below are URLs of several very reputable sites to research doctors.

- Healthgrades.com - https://www.healthgrades.com
- Care Compare - https://www.medicare.gov/care-compare/?providerType=Physician&redirect=true
- National Committee for Quality Assurance (NCQA) - https://www.ncqa.org/
- U.S. News & World Report - https://health.usnews.com/doctors
- Find Doctors and Medical Facilities - https://www.usa.gov/doctors
- American Board of Medical Specialties Verify Certification - https://www.abms.org/verify-certification

Clarify office policies

Consider:
- How well does the practice meet your needs? For instance, do you need evening or weekend appointments?
- What is the policy on medication refills?
- What is the policy on communicating test results?
- When is a reasonable expectation for the doctor to return your phone calls?
- Is the staff friendly and professional?

- How long does it typically take for a routine appointment?
- Does the office use a reputable electronic health records system?
- Does the doctor's office have a patient portal?
- Can you securely e-mail your doctor thru the portal?
- Can you book your appointments online?
- Can prescription requests be made online if you prefer?
- Is the office location acceptable to you?

The first visit is the testing ground

When you see your new doctor, take note.
- Does the doctor listen to your concerns?
- Does he explain your problem in a language you understand?
- Do you feel respected?
- Are you given ample time to address your concerns?

Selecting a doctor is a significant undertaking. Don't be in a rush. Take the time you need to research several doctors. Then narrow down the list based on your personal priorities. If, after visiting the doctor, you feel you made the wrong choice, don't worry. You can re-evaluate the others on your list or start the process anew. The important thing is that you are satisfied with a compassionate, competent doctor. This may not be a sprint. It may be a marathon.

Everyone in charge of your care may not be an MD

Everybody is familiar with the title MD, a traditional medical doctor. But you may not be aware that there's another type of physician, the doctor of osteopathic medicine, or DO. These physicians are trained differently from MDs. Their training incorporates natural and holistic healing practices. DOs are licensed physicians, like MDs. Preventive care is one particular emphasis of their education. To get into their respective schools, MDs and DOs must both pass the same medical college admissions test (MCAT). After graduation, they both enroll in an internship program. Then, they start a residency program in their chosen field, such as internal medicine. MDs and DOs may work side-by-side in the same medical practice seamlessly. The standard of care in medicine is the same whether the care is provided by an MD or DO. All medical providers, including MDs, DOs, and Advanced Practice Providers noted below must participate in ongoing medical education to help them keep current with important medical literature.

Besides physicians, there are Advanced Practice Providers, or APPs, who care for patients. These include:

- Physician assistants (PA-Cs)
- Nurse practitioners (NPs)
- Certified registered nurse anesthetists (CRNAs)
- Certified nurse midwives (CNMs)

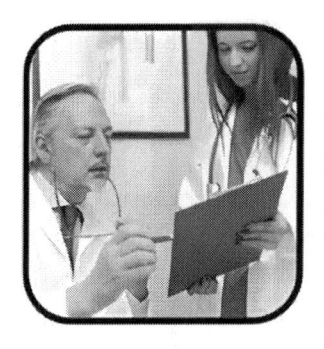

Physician assistants (PA-Cs) are licensed professionals with advanced degrees. PA-Cs are required to have national certification, the "C" in PA-C. They are educated in general medicine with a disease-centered curriculum like medical students. A PA-C may care for you at your primary care doctor's office, emergency room, and other places. State laws vary regarding the specific duties a physician assistant can have. In addition, a supervising physician oversees PA-Cs and guides their duties. They can assist in surgical procedures, prescribe medications, perform physical examinations, order and interpret diagnostic tests, and more.

Nurse practitioners (NPs) have a master's or doctorate degree and advanced clinical training beyond a typical registered nurse. Their training model is patient-centered education and practice. NPs also specialize in a specific area, such as pediatrics or family medicine. You may see a nurse practitioner at your primary care doctor's office, a hospital, and in other healthcare settings. NPs must undergo national certification too, periodic peer review, and other quality assurance evaluations. They focus on the health and well-being of the entire person. Health education, counseling, and disease prevention are areas of focus. Like physician assistants, nurse practitioners abide by the rules and regulations of their licensing state. APPs are critical to the success of the U.S. healthcare system, and their input and value are beyond profound.

> *Nurse practitioners, physician assistants and midwives are examples of Advanced Practice Providers. I've worked with several nurse practitioners and physician assistants throughout my time as a hospital doctor (hospitalist). The U.S. faces a projected shortage of between 37,800 and 124,000 physicians within 12 years. This is based on the report released by the Association of American Medical Colleges (AAMC). With the growing doctor shortage, Advanced Practice Providers do bridge this gap and allow for improved patient access to care, better patient satisfaction, and improved physician work-life balance.*
> **-Marianne Cunanan-Bush, M.D., Internist**

For simplicity, the text will call providers doctors or physicians. But know that in many instances they could be substituted for an Advanced Practice Provider.

In addition to a provider, you will need to select a pharmacy.

Choosing a pharmacy

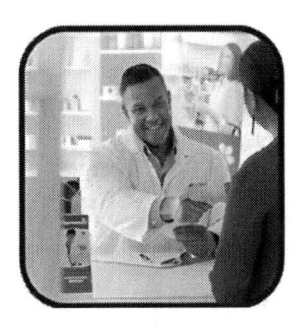

When choosing a pharmacy, there are several things to consider. Notice whether the pharmacist will answer your questions and give you good advice. Pay attention to how long you must wait to get your prescriptions filled. How friendly is the staff? In addition to the factors above, consider the following when choosing.

Accessibility

How close is the pharmacy to your home or job? You want to be sure you can get your prescriptions filled promptly. Try to select a pharmacy close to where you spend most of your time. Also, you don't want to travel a long distance to pick up your prescriptions if you get sick.

Hours

Since an emergency can occur at any time, choosing a 24/7 pharmacy will afford you the benefit of getting prescriptions filled whenever you need them. If that is not feasible, look for one with the hours that best accommodate your lifestyle.

Insurance considerations

Find out if your health insurer has a pharmacy network. This is imperative. Filling prescriptions at a convenient yet out-of-network pharmacy can be costly if you are required to use its network pharmacy. If you don't have health insurance, shop around. For example, Google "$4 medications" to find pharmacies in your area that offer a 30- day supply of many prescription drugs for $4. Make sure your physician notes on the prescription that generic substitutions are allowed. If your prescription is unavailable on a $4 prescription plan near you, Google "prescription discount cards" to learn more about other programs that may help save you money.

Check with your insurance company to see if you can receive 90-day supplies of chronic medications by mail. Having medications delivered to your door can relieve the stress of getting refills. You may even find a local pharmacy that delivers.

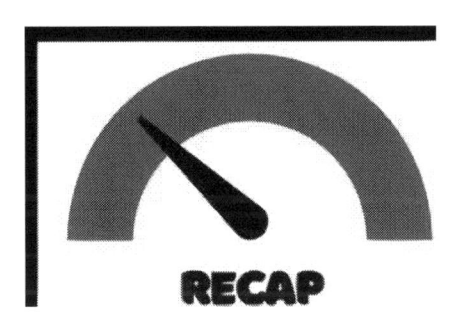

RECAP

- Your medical provider can be an MD, DO, or APP.
- Learn as much as you can about your potential doctors.
- Get recommendations for doctors.
- Find out if you need to use specific pharmacies under your insurance plan.

QUIZ

What factors should you consider when selecting a physician?

A. board certification

B. malpractice claims

C. recommendations

D. all of the above

Answer: D

Chapter 4

HEALTH INSURANCE OPTIONS

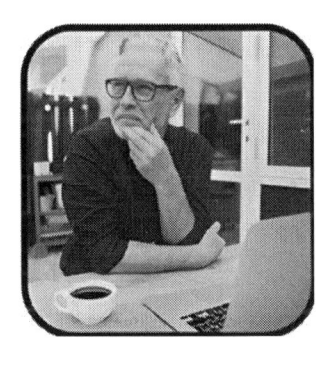

Selecting the right health insurance to cover your medical expenses is crucial. Different people have different needs, different priorities, and different budgets. They also have different expectations. There is no one-size-fits-all plan. So, unless you have an employer-sponsored health insurance which doesn't offer you any options to choose from, it's worth taking time to do your due diligence before selecting your plan.

Consider your current health status. If you need family coverage, think about how often your family members needed medical care over the past few years and how extensive it was. There is a tremendous difference between having a child with very mild asthma who routinely sees a doctor once or twice during the winter months when he catches a cold and having a child with severe asthma who has required multiple hospitalizations.

These two scenarios could result in dramatically different out-of-pocket costs based on which health insurance plan you have. When choosing a plan, consider the price of premiums, services offered, total out-of-pocket costs, your chronic conditions, and your expectation of the need for expensive medical care, such as multiple surgeries. This chapter gives you an overview of medical insurance. Health insurance is a complex topic, and different plans have their different options and caveats. Before making a final decision on which plan to pick, do detailed research into that plan and comparison shop.

Premiums

Medical plans exist to meet your needs. Insurance premiums are the fees paid to keep your policy in force. If your employer offers health insurance, you may be expected to share the cost. Luckily, many employers pay the lion's share. With employer-sponsored health insurance plans, paycheck deductions typically cover your share of the premiums.

Out-of-pocket costs

These are costs that are not covered by your health insurance. Costs may include:
- Deductibles
- Co-insurance
- Co-payments for covered services
- Charges for services that aren't covered under your plan

Not everyone has health insurance paid for or subsidized by his employer. If you are among the millions of people who purchase medical insurance on their own, there is some bright news. Your out-of-pocket expenses are capped. The Affordable Care Act established the health insurance Marketplace. This is a gateway for small businesses, families, and individuals to obtain health insurance. Healthcare.gov states that your exact out-of-pocket expenses can vary but cannot exceed set limits. In 2023, that limit is $9,100 for an individual and $18,200 for a family. In 2022, the limits were set at $8,700 and $17,400, respectively. Note these limits do not include your monthly premium, out-of-network care or services, non-covered benefits, or costs that exceed the allowed amount a provider may charge for a service. For instance, if your doctor strongly feels you need a medication not on the medication list your insurance pays for, you might pay out of pocket to get it. That preferred medication list is called a *formulary*. First, contact your insurance company to find out the steps to take to get an override to see if they will make an exception and cover that medication due to your situation. Your doctor can fill out a form explaining why you need that medication.

Deductibles

Deductibles are payments you need to make before your plan pays for your medical expenses. Plans with high deductibles have relatively low premiums. This plan is worth strongly considering if you are healthy and rarely use healthcare services. Realize if you become ill, you must pay more out of pocket before the insurance pays for your medical bills. But suppose you only visit the doctor once a year for a routine physical. There, it may be more cost-effective to take the risk of an unforeseen illness and its expenses. Only you can decide how much risk you are willing to take.

Conversely, if you choose a health plan with low deductibles, your monthly premium may be significantly higher. But if you have a chronic condition, such as diabetes or hypertension, you can anticipate regular doctor appointments. The cost of these visits and any lab tests can add up.

Co-pay

This is your contribution toward the cost of your medical treatment or service. It is a flat fee not based on the total cost of the service. For instance, each time you visit your primary care doctor, you may be asked to pay a fee of $15. Whenever you see a specialist, you may have to pay $50. And whenever you go to the ER, your co-pay may be $125. Likewise, when you pick up a prescription, you may also have to pay a co-pay. Your insurance policy should clearly explain what your co-pay is for each service.

Co-insurance

This is another form of cost-sharing but is based on a percentage of the cost of your care, as opposed to the flat-fee co-pay noted above. Your co-insurance is the percentage of the cost of medical services you are responsible for. A common co-insurance is 20%. So, for a service that costs $100, you pay $20, and your health insurance pays the remaining $80. You are sharing the cost of your care with your insurer.

Out-of-pocket medical costs can be confusing. Let's look at some examples.

Example 1

Let's say Kenneth has a health insurance plan that has an annual family deductible of $3,000 and an individual deductible of $1,000. Each person in the family would have a $1,000 deductible before the insurance pays for that individual's healthcare expenses. However, the family deductible includes the combined cost of deductibles for all family members. So, if Kenneth has a wife and four children, the family deductible of $3,000 is split between six people if needed. If they all became ill, each one would not have a $1,000 medical bill before the insurance kicks in. That would be $6,000, not the $3,000 actual combined family deductible.

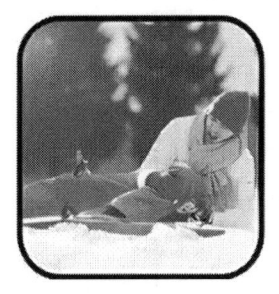

Let's take two scenarios. In the first scenario, the family goes skiing in February. Kenneth tries to impress his kids by skiing a dangerous slope he was not trained for. Sadly, Kenneth breaks a leg and has to undergo two surgeries. His first surgery costs $800. This leaves Kenneth with $200 left in his deductible ($1,000 individual deductible - $800 Kenneth pays for the surgery = $200 left in Kenneth's $1,000 individual deductible).

Scenario 1

Cost of Surgery #1 = $800

Individual Deductible Before Surgery	Family Deductible	Kenneth's Cost for Surgery #1 From Deductible	Individual Remaining Deductible After Surgery	Co-insurance of 20%
$1,000	$3,000	$800	$200	n/a
Kenneth's total cost for surgery #1: $800				

His second surgery is $700. Since he only has $200 left to pay to meet his deductible of $1,000 the insurance kicks in to help pay for the remaining $500 ($700 cost of surgery - $200 remaining deductible Kenneth needs to pay = $500 balance left to pay for the surgery). If Kenneth has a 20% coinsurance responsibility in his plan, he is responsible for 20% of that $500. So, Kenneth pays an additional $100 for the second surgery, and the insurance company pays the remaining $400.

Cost of Surgery #2 = $700

Individual Deductible Remaining Before Surgery	Family Deductible Remaining	Kenneth's Cost for Surgery #2 From Deductible	Individual Remaining Deductible After Surgery	Co-insurance of 20%
$200	$2,200	$200	$0	$500 balance X 20% co-insurance = $100 Kenneth pays for co-insurance
Kenneth's total cost for surgery #2: $200 + $100 = $300				

Scenario 2

In the second scenario, the month before the skiing trip, the entire family was driving on an icy road in a snowstorm. The SUV behind them rear-ended their car, and everyone suffered minor injuries. The combined medical bills for the family of 6 equaled $2,600. Now, there is only $400 left to pay in deductibles for the remainder of the year for the entire family ($3,000 annual family deductible - $2,600 in medical expenses = $400 remaining for the family deductible).

Family Automobile Accident Medical Expenses

~~Individual Deductible~~	Family Deductible	Family's Medical Bills	Remaining Family Deductible	Co-insurance of 20%
~~$1,000~~	$3,000	$2,600	$400	n/a
Family's total cost for medical care: $2,600				

So, when Kenneth breaks his leg skiing the following month, he is responsible for less of the cost of his surgeries. Remember, the first surgery costs $800, but he only must pay the remainder of the annual family deductible of $400 plus his 20% coinsurance ($800 cost of surgery - $400 remaining for Kenneth to pay to meet his family deductible = $400 balance due for the surgery. Now the coinsurance kicks in. Kenneth is responsible for 20% of the $400 balance, or $80. So, his total out-of-pocket expenses for the first surgery is $400 + $80 = $480. The second surgery costs $700. His deductible is met for that year, so he only must pay the 20% co-insurance cost, or $140.

Cost of Surgery #1 = $800

Remaining Individual Deductible Before Surgery (In this case, meets the remaining family deductible)	Kenneth's Cost for Surgery #1 From Deductible	Individual/Family Remaining Deductible After Surgery	Co-insurance of 20%
$400	$400	$0	$400 balance X 20% co-insurance = $80 Kenneth pays for co-insurance
Kenneth's total cost for surgery #1: $400 + $80 = 480			

Cost of Surgery #2 = $700

Remaining Individual/Family Deductible	Kenneth's Cost for Surgery #2 From Deductible	Individual/Family Remaining Deductible	Co-insurance of 20%
$0	$0	$0	$700 X 20% co-insurance = $140 Kenneth pays for co-insurance
Kenneth's total cost for surgery #2: $140			

Example 2

Cost of Medical Expenses

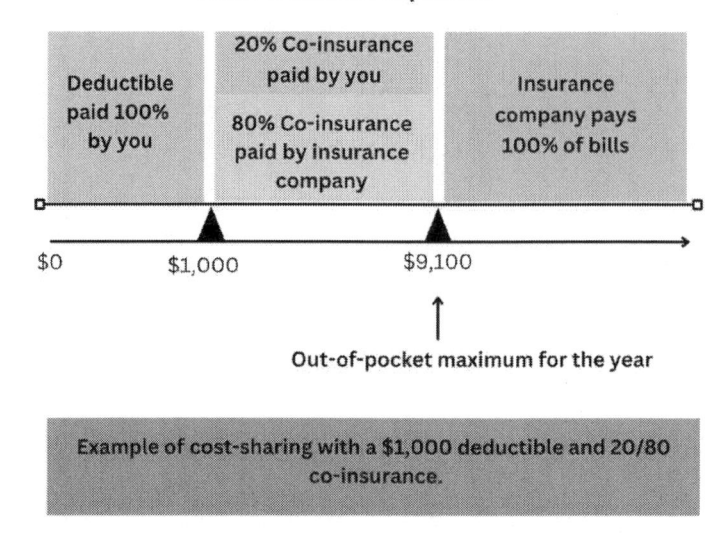

| Deductible paid 100% by you | 20% Co-insurance paid by you / 80% Co-insurance paid by insurance company | Insurance company pays 100% of bills |

$0 — $1,000 — $9,100

↑ Out-of-pocket maximum for the year

Example of cost-sharing with a $1,000 deductible and 20/80 co-insurance.

Private Health Insurance

An effective way to understand the various health plans is to consider how they are structured. Doctors contracted with a plan are called ***in-network providers***. Those without this contractual obligation are called ***out-of-network providers***. With some plans, you can visit any doctor you like; in others, you may be penalized for seeing an out-of-network provider. Below are major health plans and an explanation of how each works.

Health maintenance organizations (HMOs)

Health maintenance organizations (HMOs) are plans which limit coverage to care from a panel of doctors who contract with them. When you join, you will choose a primary care physician (PCP) or be assigned one. These doctors provide coverage to members in exchange for a monthly fee. They are the gatekeepers of our care. Your PCP refers you to specialists when needed. If you need to see a specialist, make sure your referral is approved before arriving to avoid rescheduling or having to pay out of pocket.

Care provided by an out-of-network provider is not covered unless there is an emergency or it is pre-authorized. For instance, if you need dialysis on Mondays, Wednesdays, and Fridays and plan to travel across the country to visit a relative, you can ask your HMO to approve dialysis in the area you are traveling. Different companies have different protocols, so make sure you plan for any anticipated care well before you travel.

Your PCP is also responsible for referring you for tests and procedures, such as an X-ray or lab work. This is the most cost-effective of the plans, but you may find fewer choices for doctors and more restrictions. The typical HMO does not have a deductible. An HMO may be a good choice if you don't travel frequently.

Preferred Provider Organizations (PPOs)

You'll want to consider a Preferred Provider Organization (PPO) if you prefer greater access to providers. These plans also have a network of healthcare providers who see their patients. As the name implies, they prefer you to see providers in their plan. If so, you pay less for visits. PPOs contract with medical providers, such as hospitals and doctors. They have an extensive network of participating providers. You don't need a referral to see a specialist. However, with this plan, expect higher out-of-pocket expenses.

Exclusive Provider Organizations (EPOs)

Falling somewhere between an HMO and PPO is the Exclusive Provider Organization (EPO). This plan only covers providers in-network and none out-of-network (unless it's an emergency). As with HMOs and PPOs, there are rules about obtaining healthcare, and it won't pay for your care if you don't follow its rules. Fortunately, you won't require a referral to see a specialist.

Point-of-Service (POS) plans

These plans cover in- and out-of-network providers, but you will pay less if you see a provider in-network. If you have a POS plan, you must choose an in-network PCP. Like with an HMO, the PCP issues referrals to specialists. POS plans are like PPOs in providing coverage for out-of-network providers.

HMOs, PPOs, POS, and EPO plans are all called managed care health insurance plans. They all have rules about how you receive your healthcare. The goal of managing healthcare is to keep costs down. Naturally, healthcare services should be medically necessary.

High-Deductible Health Plans (HDHPs), which may be linked to Health Savings Accounts (HSAs)

High-deductible health plans (HDHPs) can be found in HMOs and PPOs. In 2022, the IRS defined a high-deductible health plan as any plan with a deductible of $1,400+ for an individual or $2,800+ for a family. These plans obviously have a significantly higher deductible than traditional plans. But don't be in a rush to rule them out. The monthly premium is lower, often much lower.

If you have no chronic illnesses and rarely become sick, this may be the plan for you. Even if you have a chronic condition requiring regular doctor visits, it's worth considering. Pull out your calculator. Suppose your employer offers an insurance option that costs you $100 per bi-weekly pay period. There, you will pay $2,600 per year in premiums. If you have the option to select an HDHP with a $1,400 deductible and pay $20 per pay period, your premium will be $520 per year. In this scenario, an HDHP makes sense ($1,400 + $520 = $1,920 < $2,600). In this example, you would only pay the $1,400 deductible if you had at least that much in medical bills. If you only saw a doctor once or twice during the year, you would pay for less than that. In addition, you can receive preventive care at no cost to you despite not having met your deductible.

A bonus is that some HDHP plans allow you to contribute to a health savings account (HSA) via payments made by you or your employer. An HSA account allows you to make pre-tax contributions to pay for medical expenses. Money deposited into your HSA can earn interest, and your employer may match your contribution. In addition, unused HSA funds can roll over from year to year. So, while on the surface, HDHPs may cause trepidation, they have the potential to save many people a lot of money.

Government Health Insurance

Medicare and Medicaid

These are government-funded health plans with specific requirements for coverage. Each plan is designed for specific types of people. They are run by the Centers for Medicare & Medicaid Services (CMS), an agency within the U.S. Department of Health and Human Services (HHS).

Medicare

In 1965 the Medicare program was signed into law. Its original purpose was to provide medical coverage for Americans at least 65 years of age. Since its inception, the scope has expanded to include younger individuals with specific disabilities and those with End Stage Renal Disease (permanent kidney failure which requires dialysis or a kidney transplant).

Medicare coverage comprises four parts.
1. **Part A** – Hospital Insurance

Medicare Part A covers:
- inpatient care in a hospital
- skilled nursing facilities
- home health care
- nursing home care (unless custodial care is the only service you need)
- hospice care

Enrollment in Medicare Part A is considered automatic when you turn 65. While some must pay a premium for this coverage, others get Part A for free.

2. **Part B** – Medical Insurance

Medicare Part B covers:
- preventive services
- medically necessary services
- durable medical equipment (DME)
- ambulance services
- limited outpatient prescription medications
- mental health services

Medicare Part B is a voluntary program. Therefore, you must pay a monthly premium.

3. **Part C** – Medicare Advantage

Part C plans, Medicare Advantage Plans, and MA plans are all used to describe this Medicare health plan. Medicare approves private companies to offer these plans. Your plan will cover all your Part A and Part B coverage. In addition, it may provide additional coverage, including vision, dental, hearing, health, and wellness programs. Most Medicare Advantage Plans include Medicare prescription drug coverage or Part D.

4. **Part D** – Prescription Drug Coverage

Part D covers prescription medications. This benefit is available through private insurance plans approved by Medicare. All approved plans are required to cover a wide range of medicines taken by people with Medicare.

Medicaid

Medicaid is an assistance program for those with a low income. It is funded jointly by the state and federal governments. The federal government pays a specified percentage of a state's Medicaid expenditures. This program offers free or low-cost benefits to its recipients. In addition to adults with a low income, Medicaid covers children, pregnant women, those 65 years of age or older, and those with disabilities. Of note, even if your income is too high to qualify for Medicaid, your child might still qualify for the Children's Health Insurance Program (CHIP). Qualifications for CHIP vary by state. In addition, Medicaid offers a few services that Medicare does not, such as nursing home care.

It's important to note that if you qualify for both Medicaid and Medicare, you can have both. They work together to provide better health coverage while lowering costs.

Hospital Indemnity Insurance

In addition to your standard health insurance plan, you can purchase a supplemental or hospital indemnity insurance plan. Hospital bills can be exorbitant despite traditional health insurance coverage. This is where hospital indemnity insurance comes in. These plans pay you directly when hospitalized. You can use the money to pay deductibles, home care costs, or even pay for groceries. Even if you feel your plan will cover you sufficiently, planning for prolonged hospital stays and potential loss of income is essential.

Cancer Insurance and Other Supplemental Insurance

Some health conditions can devastate you and your family if you don't plan for them. Having cancer and other supplemental insurance can help you to shoulder the costs.

Cancer insurance will help cover the burden of the costs not covered by your health insurance. These insurance plans differ and can cover various medical and non-medical expenses. These plans should always be considered supplemental and not a replacement for your primary plan. Some insurance plans allow you to spend the money how you want to, while others are stricter regarding how the funds are spent.

As you can see, there are multiple types of health insurance, each with pros and cons. While you may find yourself confused by all the choices, it's worth your time to research the best option to meet your specific needs.

Insurance Denials and Appeals

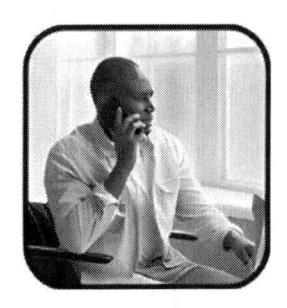

Don't be surprised if you get a denial for a health claim. This may happen before or after you've received a test or when looking for a particular treatment. This may also occur when you're looking for pre-authorization. One reason for denial may stem from your doctor recommending a test or procedure that your insurance company doesn't think you need. Medical policies guide these reasons. Each insurance company has its own internal policies. In addition, different insurance companies may reference different national guidelines to assist in their decision-making.

Before going into depth with the appeal process, it's important to note why the denial happened. The insurer may give this information in an ***explanation of benefits (EOB)*** document. This document highlights what the insurer covers and how much they cover.

Broad reasons your claim may have been denied:

- The medical service requested was deemed inappropriate or not medically necessary.
- The service requested is deemed experimental and may not have undergone scrutiny to be added to the list of covered benefits.
- Administrative errors like typos and information were entered into the computer incorrectly.
- The service requested was deemed out-of-network, and your plan has in-network providers who can provide the same service for you.

So, you are denied a service you believe you are entitled to. You can appeal the denial. The appeals process is stepwise.
- Internal appeal
- Independent external review

Internal Appeals

Start by calling the medical insurance customer service department to find out the procedure for the appeals process. Your appeal simply may involve providing additional information that was not available when the denial was issued, or it may be more complex. Each company has its own approach, so learn as much as you can about the process.

Before sending your appeal:
1. Make a copy of all documents you send.
2. If you speak to a customer care agent over the phone, get their name and a reference number for your call.
3. Follow up. If you get rejected, don't give up. Ask what the next step is to reverse the denial.

Your appeal is reviewed by a medical director at the insurance company. Your goal is to substantiate the need and prove that the insurance company should cover the denied medical service. Partnering with your doctor to appeal the denial is important. There may be treatment specifics that your doctor may have noted that will significantly assist your case. Keep all your paperwork organized, and always have your insurance information on hand when you call the insurer.

According to Healthcare.gov, your internal appeal must be completed within 30 days for a service not yet received and within 60 days for a service received. Your insurer must provide a written decision. The final determination tells you the process for requesting an external review.

Independent External Review

This is a third-party appeal that the insurance company must comply with. The independent company assesses your appeal with a doctor having appropriate qualifications to render a fair decision. It's important to note that some appeals have time constraints. Therefore, make sure you've filed all the documentation before your window of opportunity closes.

RECAP

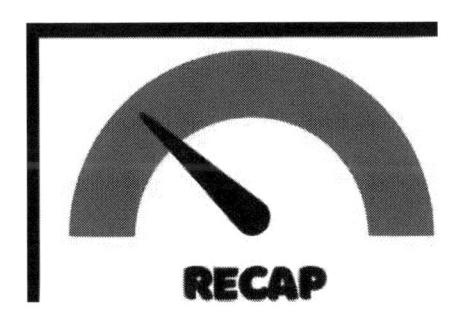

- When selecting a health insurance plan, consider your potential out-of-pocket costs.
- Know your deductible, co-insurance, and co-pay.
- Compare all the potential options in depth before deciding on a plan.
- If your insurance claim is denied, contact the company and ask about the appeals process.

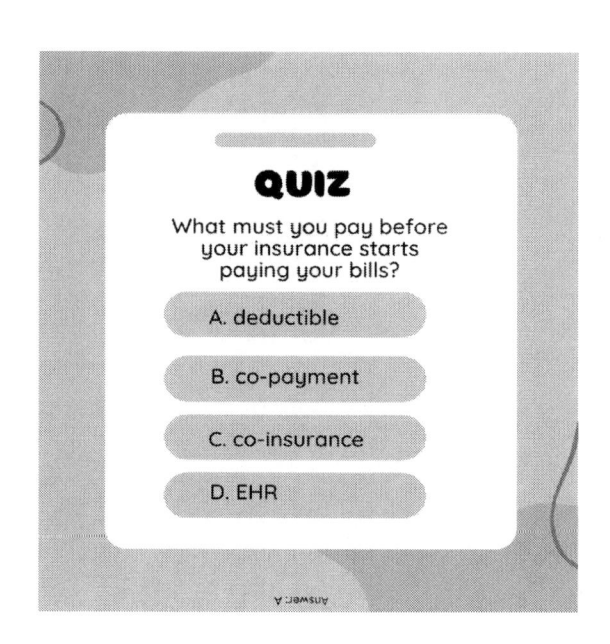

QUIZ

What must you pay before your insurance starts paying your bills?

A. deductible

B. co-payment

C. co-insurance

D. EHR

Answer: A

Chapter 5

YOUR MEDICAL RECORDS ARE VITAL

Why should you develop and maintain a personal copy of important medical records? For many reasons. We first need to put things in perspective to understand how imperative this task is. Most Americans are aware of the decades-long debate over health care reform. Many questions remain. Viable solutions to providing top-notch health care to all Americans are evading even the most brilliant experts. Insurance companies and physicians are busily trying innovative new approaches to optimize health care in the face of never-ending unique, often unpredictable challenges. Just look at how the COVID-19 pandemic devastated our healthcare system. Multitudes of elective surgeries were cancelled. Patients could not get in to see their doctors. These things are two of a multitude of challenges brought on by the virus. Who knows what's next with COVID-19? Who knows if another pandemic is on the horizon?

Even at baseline, America's healthcare industry is in a state of flux, born out of desperation to improve affordability while maintaining access to exceptional health care. Undoubtedly, the desire to put a lid on skyrocketing health care costs was a significant impetus to this movement. According to the Centers for Medicare & Medicaid Services (CMS), National Health Expenditures (NHE) grew 9.7% in 2020 to $4.1 trillion. This accounted for 19.7% of the Gross Domestic Product (GDP). In addition, between 2019-2028, national health spending is projected to grow by approximately 5.4 percent annually, reaching $6.2 trillion by 2028. CMS also projects National Health Expenditures to grow 1.1 percentage points faster than the yearly GDP over the same time. Where will it end? Who can afford quality healthcare if prices continue to rise at this rate?

In this era of uncertainty and mistrust, it is crucial for healthcare consumers to be empowered to weather the storm. We can no longer afford to have blind faith in the potentially life-altering decisions made by others, no matter how brilliant or noble they may be. It is time for Americans to take an unprecedented step toward actively participating in their own health care. Everyone must stand up and participate in the crucial health care decisions that affect their lives.

America has traditionally had a paternalistic healthcare system. Physicians have taken the lead, and patients have been expected to follow blindly, much like small children innately trust and obey their parents. However, in contrast to a few decades ago, when a patient often had the same doctor for 20 or 30 years, patients today frequently move from doctor to doctor based on which insurance company has offered their employer the best rates and which doctors participate in their plans.

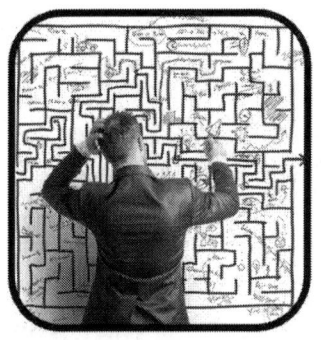

This lack of continuity of care throws yet another level of complexity into the already complicated maze of a health system. For example, prior records are often vital in helping physicians optimally care for patients. However, the new physician must get signed consent from the patient to obtain those records. The release is then sent to prior physicians. Then the wait begins. When time is of the essence, even two weeks can seem like a lifetime. Therefore, it is often in your best interest for the physician to simply order the tests she feels are necessary. Often, these tests were already done.

Frequently, patients cannot remember enough information about prior physicians to request their old records. And if that physician is deceased or retired, obtaining old records may be virtually impossible. The result is that expensive, sometimes painful tests are repeated, delaying optimal treatment and increasing medical costs. But when a patient is suffering and old records are not readily available, what choice does a physician have?

There is yet another twist to our already complicated health system. To balance reimbursements received from insurance companies against escalating practice expenditures, physicians may need to see a high number of patients each day. Within this quota of patients, there will invariably be new and established patients, routine patients, and very sick patients. Many patients and patient problems can be encountered on any day.

The purpose of this chapter is not to make you a medical expert but to empower you to play an active role in your own health. It does this by teaching you the fundamentals needed to develop a dynamic personal copy of your medical records. Your document will not be as detailed as your physician's record. If it were, you probably could not understand it. Your copy will focus on the essential facts that will help you receive prompt and accurate medical treatment.

Organizing this crucial information is as important as obtaining it. Physicians are busy. Chances are when you schedule a doctor's appointment, you will be scheduled for a 15- or 30-minute slot, depending on your visit's anticipated complexity level. If you bring in a stack of medical records two inches thick, your doctor cannot read much of it during your visit. Instead, she will skim the surface with hopes of finding time later to read it in its entirety. Remember, however, that she may see hundreds of patients each week and an unending mound of administrative work to get to when time allows. You can help her tremendously by organizing your records in a concise, easy-to-read manner.

Since the days of the family doctor seeing a patient from delivery to retirement are all but gone, a personal copy of your health records is an absolute must. Communication with future physicians can be accomplished without the untimely delays of waiting weeks or longer to receive prior records from another physician - if that doctor is still accessible. Even if a doctor you saw years ago is still available, your old records may not be. They may have been destroyed and obliterated with zero chance of recovery. Physicians are only required to keep old medical records for a specific period, often 7 years, but this can vary from state to state.

You can see why having a personal copy of your health records is crucial. Who can predict whether diagnoses and test results from the past may be pertinent to the future? But, more importantly, why risk it? Creating a personal copy of health records can be simple yet potentially lifesaving.

> *Everyone involved in the care of elderly patients should keep an updated list of their medicines in the Notes section of their cell phone. When a patient requires an interaction with any medical provider (whether in the ER or office) this should be the master list to be sure their medicines are reconciled properly and efficiently.*
>
> *It takes time to contact doctors' offices to get the medication list from previous records. Patients often write a list of their medications on papers with words scratched out and wrong doses listed. Access to a clean, up-to-date, easily accessible list is best achieved and archived using the Notes app on a cell phone. Finally, all patients should ask to take a picture of their last EKG using their cell phone and store it in this section of their phone for easy accessibility as well.*
>
> **-Marc Okun, M.D. Cardiologist**

Our bodies don't read medical textbooks, so you must know your body well. For instance, a slightly low blood calcium level does not cause symptoms in most people. But in a small minority, uncomfortable symptoms occur at levels most people tolerate seamlessly. Discuss any abnormal lab results with your doctor. Your symptoms may be a complete coincidence and have no clinical significance. But ask your doctor if she thinks your symptoms are related to the minor lab abnormality noted. Reinforcement from a healthcare provider will increase the likelihood that there is a correlation.

However, even if your doctor does not think there is an association, document your symptoms anyway. Note that your doctor did not believe there was a causal relationship with the lab abnormality. Suppose you experience similar symptoms in the future with a similarly "slightly abnormal" lab result. There, it is more likely that the association is real. You must understand your medical issues to explain them to future providers.

> *Check in with your body. When it tells you something, listen to it.*
>
> **-Dipa Mair, MSN, RN**

While you may rely on a patient portal or mobile app to keep track of your records, you still need a physical copy. You may change insurance companies and lose access to the patient portal. The mobile device that houses your app may accidentally fall in the bathtub. Ouch!

You need to know specifics about your past medical history for several reasons. Always write down the precise medical terms for your illnesses, and do not be satisfied knowing you have "some kidney or lung problem." Exact information empowers you to communicate optimally with future healthcare providers and aid them in treating your condition promptly and effectively. Many diseases have well-recognized complications or a predictable course. By knowing the exact names of prior diagnoses, your doctor will be much better equipped to diagnose any future problems attributable to that illness. A treatment that otherwise may have been rendered may be adjusted or avoided.

For instance, Goodpasture's syndrome is a disease that commonly affects the lungs and kidneys. Suppose all you remember about your condition is that a prior physician told you something was wrong with your kidneys. There, future physicians will be at a disadvantage in treating you. Goodpasture's syndrome is a rare disease, and routine screening lab tests do not confirm this diagnosis. Furthermore, the esoteric tests that diagnose Goodpasture's syndrome can be costly, so a physician will not order them unless he has a strong suspicion of this disease.

A "kidney problem" can be a mild congenital abnormality of no clinical significance. However, it could also be a rapidly progressing life-threatening disease. With Goodpasture's syndrome, both the kidneys and lungs are affected. Specifically, there is the potential for life- threatening bleeding in the lungs. However, you may not have severe lung symptoms and not tell your doctor about any new breathing problems, particularly if you have another lung disease, such as emphysema. You may attribute any lung symptoms to this. Let's say all your physician knows is that you have some obscure history of an undefined kidney problem. The initial screening blood work confirms some type of kidney disease. Your doctor may focus a lot of unnecessary time and money on determining its cause. But remember, there are many kidney problems.

This can be even further obscured if you also have another disease that commonly leads to kidney problems, such as diabetes or hypertension. In such instances, your kidney abnormalities may be chalked up to a common cause of kidney disease, and no additional tests will be run. Alternatively, a basic kidney work-up is initiated. Still, without further crucial history from you, esoteric, expensive tests are not included because they are deemed of little value.

The following are some of the common symptoms experienced by a person with Goodpasture's syndrome and a partial list of other potential causes of those symptoms.

Symptoms seen with Goodpasture's syndrome	Other potential causes of these symptoms
Nausea/vomiting	- inflammation of the stomach lining (gastritis) - inflammation of the pancreas (pancreatitis) - Inflammation of the esophagus (esophagitis) - gallstones/gallbladder inflammation - medication - heart disease - irritable bowel syndrome (IBS) - gastroenteritis ("a stomach bug") - bowel obstruction - ulcers - pregnancy - and many more
Blood in the urine	- a bladder infection - kidney stones - trauma - inflammation of the blood vessels in the kidneys - tumors
Cough	- bronchitis - pneumonia - asthma - gastroesophageal reflux disease (GERD) - common cold - allergies

	• medication side effects
	• lung cancer
	• influenza
Fatigue	• depression
	• anemia
	• viral syndrome
	• underactive thyroid
	• some muscle diseases
	• sleep apnea
	• medications
Anemia	• iron deficiency
	• vitamin B12 deficiency
	• monthly menstrual cycles
	• slow/intermittent internal bleeding
	• inherited anemia
	• some chronic diseases
	• bone marrow disorders
	• cancer

You can easily see how naming one or two of these symptoms is enough to send your doctor on a wild goose chase without ever even considering Goodpasture's syndrome. He may undertake an extensive, very expensive, and time-consuming workup that may never reveal the underlying diagnosis. However, simply relaying the name Goodpasture's syndrome would put you on the road to more accurate diagnoses of future associated conditions. The appropriate treatment will be forthcoming quicker.

For instance, the average person who develops a simple bout of acute bronchitis may occasionally cough up sputum with streaks of blood. This would not cause much alarm for the physician. However, suppose a patient with known Goodpasture's syndrome complained of bloody sputum. There, the doctor may be much more aggressive in ordering tests to determine the exact cause, realizing that that patient is at risk of having a potentially severe lung hemorrhage.

You should never assume that when a doctor says he is going to "run tests," he will find out everything he needs to know about a disease he is unaware of. For example, there are many blood tests that help diagnose different diseases. Some are routine screening tests, such as a metabolic profile (blood chemistry test) or complete blood count (CBC). Others are expensive, esoteric tests that may need to be sent to a reference lab hundreds of miles away because no local laboratory can perform them.

In this era of financial constraints, many insurance companies will not pay for tests considered "medically unnecessary." For example, let's say you go to a doctor's office for an annual exam. You had no symptoms of any ailment. Based on your insurance, you may not be able to have "routine" lab tests done unless you were willing to pay for them yourself.

Getting back to Goodpasture's syndrome, the blood tests that help diagnose this condition are expensive. Since this is a rare disease, the expense of running these tests routinely cannot be justified. Therefore, as with all other diseases, you would be best served by having specific details about your medical history for future healthcare workers to review. Goodpasture's syndrome is a serious condition, and while you likely would not forget a condition this severe, it was chosen for illustrative purposes.

In addition, you should not only write the names of all diagnosed conditions but also chart how these illnesses were diagnosed. For instance, if you were diagnosed with ulcers, was this diagnosis confirmed by an upper GI (gastrointestinal) test in the X-ray department? Did you undergo an upper endoscopy (also called an esophagogastroduodenoscopy [EGD]) done by a gastroenterologist? Or was this simply a presumptive diagnosis based on the history you gave the physician? Suppose you suffer from stomach pain and respond to agents that decrease acid in the stomach. That does not automatically mean you have ulcers. You may have had gastritis (inflammation of the stomach lining) or some condition unrelated to acid in the stomach. That your symptoms resolved on treatment that blocks stomach acid may have been coincidental.

In the future, if a similar condition arises, it would be good for your physician to know how the diagnosis was initially made. If the diagnosis of an ulcer was made solely on clinical grounds (your history), it may behoove you to have an upper endoscopy. During this procedure, a biopsy can be taken of the stomach lining. Helicobacter pylori is a type of bacteria associated with peptic ulcer disease. By eradicating it with medication, your risk of developing future ulcers will be decreased significantly. Since a complicated ulcer can lead to potentially life-threatening internal bleeding and severe pain, it would be prudent to treat it optimally. There are other tests to detect Helicobacter pylori as well. Still, it is good to chart the specifics of the diagnosis, such as "diagnosed by Dr. Wesley Matthews by an upper endoscopy (EGD) at Kensington Hospital, in Memphis, TN in 2021." Charts are provided for download to help you create your medical record.

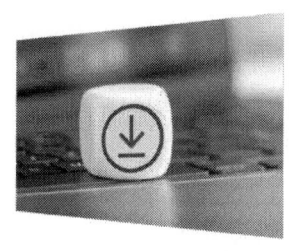

Go to: https://www.patientempowerment101.com/my-records to download charts.

Creating a personal health record is quite simple. Start by buying a 3-ring binder and dividers with tabs you can customize. Expect to pick up more than one package of dividers to keep track of all the sections.

Next, create these sections:
- Emergency contact information

- Insurance information
- Medical providers
    - PCPs and specialists
    - Non-physician providers, such as chiropractors
- Chronic medical conditions (such as diabetes)
- Acute medical conditions (such as the flu)
- Appointments
- Medications
- Pharmacy information
- Mini-medical record (keep a copy in your wallet)
- Medication allergies/intolerances
- Hospitalizations
- Family history
- Surgeries and procedures
- Social history
- Immunizations/ health screenings
- Health logs; blood pressure, blood sugar, and cholesterol
- Personal health goals; exercise log and dietary habits
- Correspondence
- Test results
- Advance care planning
- Miscellaneous (such as information from home health agencies you have used)

Below you will find information about various components of your personal health record and sample charts. You may also download these fillable charts as noted above. Create a desktop folder and save blank copies. You may also want to save the forms you filled in as another backup for your records. You can place them in the Miscellaneous section of your binder. The charts have limited space, but you can jot down any notes and details on the back of the page.

Emergency Contact Information

It is important to always have your emergency contact information available. This is not just for medical providers. It will help you too. Some people keep phone numbers in their cell phone and never memorize them. If the battery dies or the phone is lost, that could put you in quite a predicament. There may come a time when a doctor needs to reach a close family member quickly. That's not the time to realize you cannot reach your family or close contact. Use this chart to document multiple contacts. Your mini-medical record chart includes abbreviated emergency contact information and you should keep a copy in your wallet.

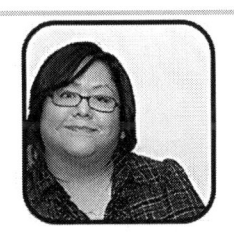

emergency contacts

Name	Relationship	Contact Info	Notes

Insurance Information

Take your insurance card with you to every medical visit. Even if the office already has your insurance information on file, they may need to make a quick call to clarify an issue. To avoid unexpected medical bills and potentially embarrassing situations, read through your policy's provisions. Many doctors' offices request payment when services are rendered. The check-out window is no place to discover that you have a $500 deductible, especially if you only have $5 in your pocket. After your deductible has been met, know what percentage of your medical bills is your responsibility. Likewise, know your co-payment for office and emergency room visits. Finally, be prepared to pay your coinsurance when asked.

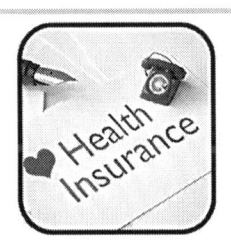

health insurance

Insurance name	
Member ID	
Group #	
RxBIN	
RxGRP	
Contact info	
Notes	

Insurance name	
Member ID	
Group #	
RxBIN	
RxGRP	
Contact info	
Notes	

Insurance name	
Member ID	
Group #	
RxBIN	
RxGRP	
Contact info	
Notes	

My Providers

Document all your medical providers, whether they are physicians or not. Include primary care doctors, specialists, and other providers, such as chiropractors. Over time it's easy to forget names. This can be problematic if you need to contact a prior doctor to get old records.

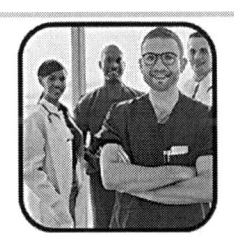

my doctors

Doctor's name	Specialty	Contact info	Date of 1st Appt

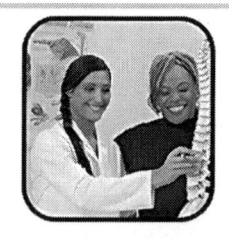

non-physician providers

Doctor's Name	Specialty	Contact Info	Date of 1st Appt

Chronic Medical Conditions

As noted, knowing the specific names of all your diagnoses is crucial. Over the course of years, you may be diagnosed with a variety of conditions. Some are chronic, such as high blood pressure. Others are acute, short-lived issues, such as the flu. Regardless of the type, thoroughly document your medical diagnoses and try to commit each name to memory.

Use the back of the form to jot down specific details and other information deemed important, such as tests used to diagnose a condition. It's also worth noting differing opinions from two doctors regarding a condition. There are many issues that may be worthwhile documenting, but there is not enough space in a chart to write down everything of importance.

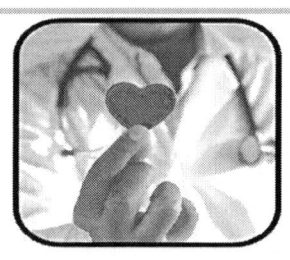

chronic medical conditions

Medical Diagnosis	Date Diagnosed	Diagnosing Doctor	Notes

Acute Medical Conditions

Naturally, from time to time, you will get sick. We all do. Jot down your diagnoses to keep track of which condition you had and when. If your doctor sees a trend, such as five urinary tract infections in one year, it may have implications for future treatment options and diagnostic tests.

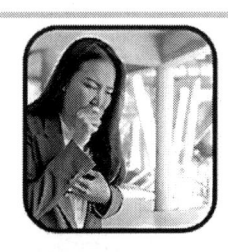

acute medical conditions

Medical Diagnosis	Date Diagnosed	Diagnosing Doctor	Notes

Appointments

Everyone forgets appointments occasionally. But when the appointment is for a health-related issue, it could have significant ramifications. First, keeping up with all issues pertaining to your health is important, even if it's just a routine follow-up visit for a chronic problem. In addition, if you do not cancel an appointment within a certain cancellation window, you may be responsible for a monetary fine. Also, remember someone else could have potentially been put into the appointment slot you missed. The bottom line is that you should document your upcoming appointments. But there is more. Jot down important issues around the appointment, such as the reason for the visit and the diagnosis given. The accompanying chart gives additional details of what's important to note.

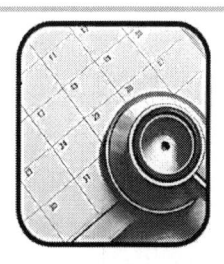

appointments

Date			
Reason for appt			
Doctor			
Specialty			
Tests ordered			
Test results			
Diagnosis			
New prescriptions			
Follow-up needed (if any)			
Notes			

Date			
Reason for appt			
Doctor			
Specialty			
Tests ordered			
Test results			
Diagnosis			
New prescriptions			
Follow-up needed (if any)			
Notes			

Medications

During your lifetime, you'll take various medications, even if you do not have any chronic illnesses. It is unrealistic to think that you will recall all their names. Still, it would be beneficial for you to keep a record of the medications your doctors prescribe. Note whether they worked for you and whether they caused any unpleasant side effects.

Suppose you have an illness for which your doctor has tried 4 or 5 medications before finding the one that works right for you. There, you need to remember that specific drug so you don't have to go through another round of trial and error if you develop similar symptoms in the future.

> *Medication adherence is an intricate global issue faced by patients and clinicians. Non-adherence has significant economic and therapeutic consequences affecting the overall quality of life. Medication adherence is a complex behavioral process affected by numerous factors. There are various tools and methods to measure and aid in medication adherence.*
>
> *However, there is no "one size fits all" solution to improve adherence. Initiation of medication adherence starts when a prescription is generated.*
> - *Phase 1 is obtaining the medication. Barriers in Phase 1 include in-person factors (transportation, caregiver issues, attitude) and mail-order factors (patient is on an unstable regimen).*
> - *Phase 2 is organizing multiple medications to manageable adherence.*
> - *Phase 3 consists of problems with taking the medications for various reasons. The barriers in Phase 3 are numerous. Some examples include:*
>   - *expense of chronic medications*
>   - *lack of patient education regarding the importance of ongoing compliance*
>   - *patient believes they are experiencing an "adverse event"*
>   - *patient does not feel any differently on the medication*
>   - *inability to take the medication*
>   - *lack of support for ongoing compliance.*
>
> *All lead to potential discontinuation. Therefore, improving medication adherence depends on the underlying problem based on the above. Solutions can range from simplistic pill boxes to sophisticated drug delivery systems. One Size Does Not Fit All.*
>
> **-Erkan Hassan, Pharm.D., FCCM**

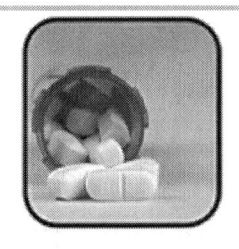

medications

Medication Brand Name/ Generic Name	Prescribing Doctor	Dosage and Frequency	Reason for Taking

Pharmacy Information

Keep track of the pharmacies you use to get your prescriptions filled. With large chains and smaller, locally owned pharmacies, it's easy to forget which pharmacy you used for which prescription. It's best to use the same pharmacy for all your prescriptions, but sometimes that is not realistic. You may move too far away to continue to use the same pharmacy. Your insurance may change, and your pharmacy might not be on their preferred pharmacy list.

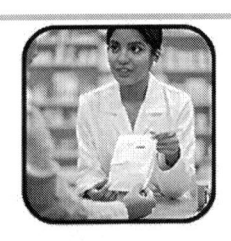

my pharmacies

Pharmacy Name	Contact Info	Hours	Notes

Mini-Medical Record

Naturally, you will not always have a detailed copy of health records with you, but you can keep the most important information in your wallet. That way, you can quickly pull it out in an unforeseen emergency and give your medical providers instant access to vital information about your health. Remember to keep it updated. Jot the dates updated at the top of the form, so it will be clear to others just how recent this important document is.

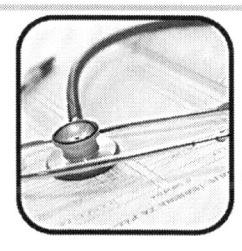

My Mini Medical Record

My Name:		Emergency Contact Name:
My Phone#:		Relationship:
		Phone #1:
My Doctor's Name:		Phone #2:
Phone #:		Other info:
Pharmacy Name:		
Phone #:		

My Chronic Conditions	My Medication Allergies/Intolerances	
	Medication Name	Reaction

My Medications			My Surgeries
Medication Name	Dosage	Instructions	

Drug Allergies and Intolerances

When you have an adverse drug reaction, document it. Be specific. Do not automatically consider yourself allergic to medication just because it made you feel funny. For example, if codeine in a cough syrup makes you feel woozy, this may be because codeine is a narcotic. It makes a lot of people feel that way. Yet, that differs from a true codeine allergy. An actual allergic reaction to a drug can be fatal. So, it is essential to specify the type of reaction you have to any medication.

A more common example is that aspirin frequently causes stomach upset. Many drug manufacturers have developed coated aspirin to decrease this common side effect. However, stomach upset after taking aspirin is not a true aspirin allergy. People truly allergic to aspirin can die if they use aspirin products. We know that some people can die if stung by a bee. A true aspirin allergy is similar.

Before you claim to be allergic to a medication, speak with your doctor. There may come a time that you need that medication, or one like it, to save your life. If your doctor thinks you are allergic to that drug, you will not get it. Instead, you will be prescribed the second most effective drug for that situation. You want the best treatment possible, not the second best. Don't wait until you are in an emergency to clarify your allergies. You may not be able to communicate effectively then, and your relatives may have to relay your medical history to the best of their ability. But what if they don't know the answers?

Aspirin has been shown to decrease the chance of dying from an acute heart attack. It is one of the first medications an emergency room physician orders if he thinks you may have this potentially life-threatening condition. If your close relatives tell the emergency room physician you are allergic to aspirin, you may not get it. You can see that what may seem trivial may prove dangerous to your health.

There are numerous equally important scenarios involving a wide range of other medications. So, remember to record your reaction when you have an adverse response to a medication. Many drugs have copycat substitutes with similar chemical structures but different names. You may be allergic to these substitutes too. Knowing the exact names of medications that cause adverse effects can avoid a potentially dangerous situation.

Finally, reviewing your medication history can give your healthcare providers insight into previously diagnosed conditions, even while awaiting old records from a prior doctor. Some medications are classically used for a specific condition, and simply knowing what drugs you were on in the past may benefit your current and future physicians.

Just as importantly, take medications as prescribed. It's natural to occasionally forget to take a pill or take it later than usual. But if this becomes habitual, you may be in an emergency. To help you keep up with your medications, you can pick up an inexpensive pill box at your local pharmacy. These boxes can be basic, with a single compartment each day. This may be all you need if you take only one medication or if you take more than one medication but take all your pills simultaneously each day.

But they can be fancier. For example, you can buy pill boxes with 2, 3, or even 4 slots per day for medications requiring multiple daily doses. You can even find boxes with 28 slots for 4 weeks' worth of pills.

Tell your doctor if she prescribed medication not within your budget. There are usually cheaper alternatives. Infrequently, a specific medication is strongly recommended, and there are no viable alternatives. This may be the case with drugs that are new to the market and have no generic option. Fortunately, in most cases, your doctor can prescribe a different, less expensive medication. While it may not be a 100% substitute for the more costly drug, it may be a close alternative.

Also, some pharmaceutical companies sponsor Patient Assistance Programs, which provide discounted or free medications and co-pay programs. There are guidelines for inclusion in these programs geared to help those with low income or those uninsured or underinsured. Ask your doctor if the medication he strongly feels you need may be obtainable through this program. Also ask if he has samples of new medications to see if they agree with you. This may also save you money.

Don't get overwhelmed with the number of potential side effects of a medication. Every medication has the POTENTIAL to do harm, though this is the exception and not the rule. Even over-the-counter medicines, vitamins, and "all-natural" supplements can be problematic for some. For example, iron constipates some people, but a person with anemia may simply need a different formulation or dosing schedule to benefit from its potential to increase the much-needed number of red blood cells. Likewise, aspirin can upset your stomach or even cause internal bleeding. Still, it is well tolerated by most people when taken as directed (and not on an empty stomach). The list goes on and on.

If you take your bottles with you to each visit, your provider may see you have missed several doses. Alternatively, based on the day the prescription was filled, a simple pill count will tell you whether you missed any doses or took extra ones. For instance, if you had a 30-day prescription filled on March 1st, and on April 1st, there are pills left in the bottle, you know you missed some doses.

Resist the urge to reuse the same pill bottle by dumping the newly prescribed pills into an old pill bottle. There are several potential problems with this. First, you may accidentally pour in the wrong medication. Next, suppose the pills look different from the last refill, as can occur if a different company is now supplying your pharmacy with that generic medication. There, you can get confused and think you are taking the wrong medication, especially if you have any pills left over from the prior prescription.

Ask your doctor for a 90-day prescription to decrease the chance you will run out and not get around to getting a refill on time. Another perk is that 90-day supplies may save you money. If you use a mail-order pharmacy, make sure you have a local prescription of vital medications, even if only for a short supply. Then, if your medication arrives late in the mail, you will not find yourself in a potentially unsafe situation.

Consider using technology to help you remember to take your medications. Countless people have downloaded one of the numerous medication reminder apps on their smartphones. Ask your doctor or pharmacist for a recommendation or…Google it. Check out current customers' reviews and review several apps before deciding which one is right for you.

Online stores have a wide range of medication reminder options. You can find a recordable alarm clock, locked automatic pill dispensers, a vibrating watch, automatic pill dispensers, and much more. In addition, you can make very simple reminders for yourself or for those with cognitive issues or dementia. This can make a caregiver's task much easier.

You'll get to know your pharmacists if you use the same pharmacy for all your medication. You can also rest assured that since all your medication is on one computer, there is less chance of an error. Many computers have software that automatically alerts the pharmacist if she tries to fill a prescription that will interact with one you already have. When your pharmacist is alerted to potential danger, she can call your provider and notify him of the concerns. If the possible reaction is minor, your provider may tell the pharmacist to fill the prescription. He may feel if you take it, the risk of harm is far less than the risk of harm if you don't and become sicker. Whatever the case, if your pharmacist knows everything you are taking, you are better off.

You can also ask her about over-the-counter medications and supplements you are considering purchasing. You may even want to ask your pharmacist, now a trusted friend, if the medication has a less expensive alternative. Once you develop a relationship with your pharmacist, you will feel more comfortable asking any medication question.

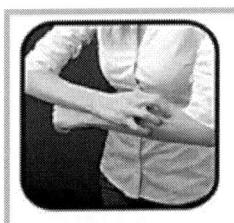

allergic reactions

Medication Brand Name	Medication Generic Name	Allergic Reaction (Be specific, i.e., hives or upset stomach.)	Date of Reaction

Hospitalizations

A stay in the hospital can be very anxiety-provoking. You will meet a host of new doctors, nurses, and other healthcare professionals. Keeping up with everyone's name can be challenging. Request a copy of the ***hospital discharge summary***. This summary summarizes why you went to the hospital, important tests and their results, and treatments rendered. It should also include key consultants on your case. Discharge medications, follow-up instructions, test results pending at discharge, and other important information is also included. Before discharge, ask about the steps to take to get a copy of your discharge summary. This document gives a great deal of information about your stay and is invaluable.

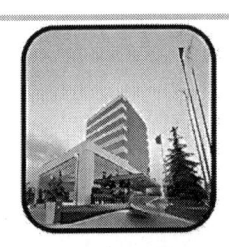

hospitalizations

Hospital Name	Major Diagnosis	Primary Doctor	Dates

Family History

The list of diseases that can run in families is exhaustive. Inheritable diseases may be passed down through the generations in various ways. Humans have 46 chromosomes in each body cell (except the eggs and sperm, each of which has 23). Each chromosome has many different regions, called genes, which "code" for everything from how tall you will become to your eye color. Our genetic map is in our chromosomes.

Your mother donated 23 chromosomes by her egg, and your father donated a matching 23 chromosomes in his sperm. Although specific genes on these chromosomes vary significantly from person to person, each chromosome from one parent pairs up with a matching chromosome from the other parent. Each complementary pair makes up a set of chromosomes. Consequently, we have 23 sets of chromosomes, for a total of 46 individual chromosomes.

Your genetic make-up may put you at risk of developing certain diseases. It's important to know what medical conditions run in your family so you can do all you can to decrease your risk, or at least minimize the dangers. For instance, if you know diabetes runs in your family, you can work hard to maintain a healthy weight, eat a healthy diet, and exercise. Doing these things can go a long way in helping optimize your health.

FAMILY TREE

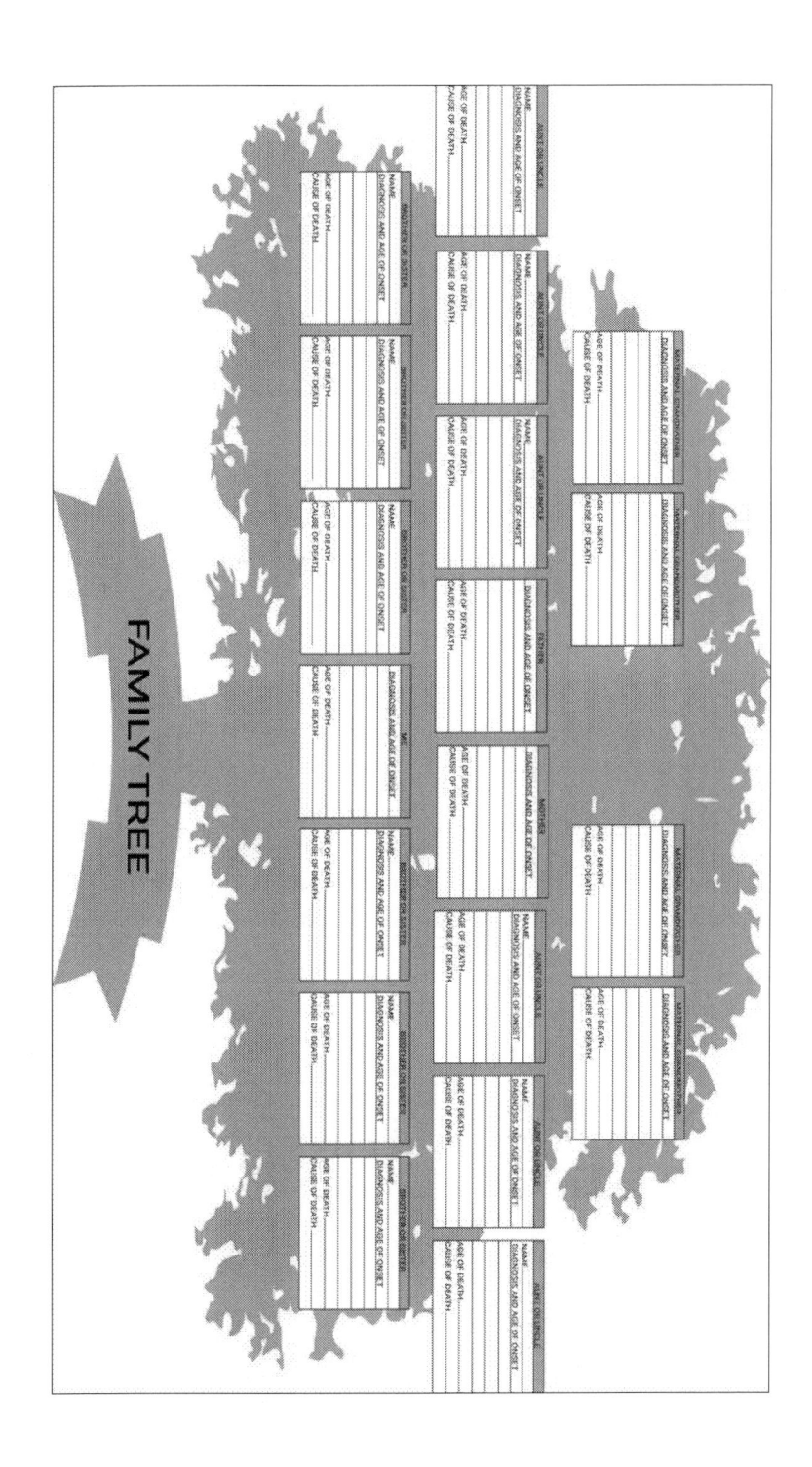

Surgeries and Procedures

Your surgical history is critical. Document every surgical procedure you have, no matter how minor. Note the exact reason for the surgery. This may seem obvious, but really, it is not. For instance, you may have your gallbladder removed because you had an inflamed gallbladder due to gallstones. Alternatively, you could have had the same surgery because your gallbladder did not effectively move bile into the bile ducts. In the first case, **cholecystitis** is the diagnosis. In the second, it is **biliary dyskinesia**. On the back of your log of surgeries, record any surgical complications you may have had.

Interestingly, some people who have undergone surgery can only discuss it superficially. For instance, some women who had hysterectomies many years prior forget whether their ovaries were removed or left intact. If one ovary was removed, they might not recall which one. If they later develop abnormal pain or a mass in their pelvic region, it would help to know what organs are in that region as soon as possible. The more tests that need to be ordered, the longer the delay in diagnosis and the more expensive the overall process.

In addition to surgeries, document your procedures, such as colonoscopies. This is also vital health information. Adding this information will give a more complete picture of your medical care.

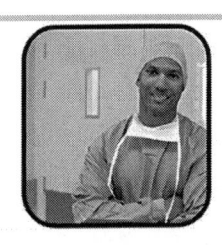

my surgeries

Surgery	Name of Surgeon	Facility	Date

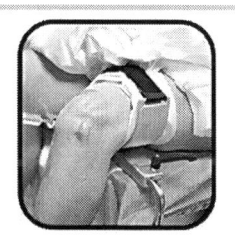

my procedures

Procedure	Name of Doctor	Facility	Date

> *You have the right to, and you must know what, when, how, and why regarding your therapy and who and why they are involved. You must understand the benefits, risks, and all outcomes with and without the treatment. Be confident and ask, enquire, or request a second opinion if necessary. Only you can be your biggest advocate.*
>
> **-M. Cornelious Musara, M.D., FACS, Surgeon**

Social History

Your social history matters. Don't worry. It is not an assessment of how many parties you go to or how active you are on social media. This is another integral part of your overall health picture. Your current and past habits and exposures may put you at risk for specific medical conditions. This is why it is so valuable.

Social history consists of several key elements. First, your ***tobacco history*** is vital. Cigarette smoking is the leading cause of preventable death in America. It is associated with premature heart attacks, chronic bronchitis and emphysema (COPD), cancer of the mouth, throat, esophagus, lungs, pancreas, and bladder, and other diseases.

The death toll attributable to smoking tobacco is staggering. According to the Centers for Disease Control and Prevention (CDC), approximately one in every five deaths in America is linked to cigarette smoking. That's over 480,000 preventable deaths each year! If you were told that every day in America, three 747 jets would crash, killing everyone on board, would you ever fly again? Probably not. Yet even that gruesome number is far less than those who die from cigarette smoking.

Smokers have a life expectancy of at least 10 years shorter than nonsmokers. Even those exposed to secondhand smoke have a higher likelihood of dying prematurely. Over 40,000 annual deaths are associated with secondhand smoke. Heart attacks and lung cancer are the primary culprits. But there is good news. Smokers who quit before turning 40 have close to a 90% decreased risk of dying from a smoking-related disease. If you are much older, throwing out your cigarettes is still a benefit. This is a book about self-empowerment and few things you do can affect your health as much as smoking cessation.

Many people think lung cancer is the primary danger of smoking cigarettes. However, it may surprise you that most deaths related to cigarette smoking are attributed to heart attacks, the number one killer in America. Many people have kicked the habit and may not realize that their smoking history is still important. For example, when asked, "Do you smoke cigarettes?" you may truthfully answer no. But suppose you smoked two packs of cigarettes per day for 15 years but quit two years ago. There, there is still a chance that your doctor may diagnose some smoking-related illness in the future.

Let's say you are 41 years old and have no family history of early heart disease. However, you already have advanced heart disease due to a long history of smoking cigarettes. It may be several years before you have any significant symptoms. Still, you could suffer a massive heart attack at 44 or 45 due to the damage that began years ago. So remember, when your doctor asks you if you smoke, be precise. For instance, you can say, "No, I have never used any form of tobacco product." Or you can say, "Yes, I smoked about one and a half packs of cigarettes a day for 20 years, but I stopped six years ago to live a more healthful lifestyle. Now I smoke five or six cigars a week." Your accuracy can go a long way in helping your doctor estimate your risk of future diseases.

Physicians often quantify a person's smoking history in terms of **pack years.** Pack years can easily be derived by multiplying the approximate number of packs of cigarettes smoked per day by the number of years you smoked. For example, if you smoked one pack per day for 20 years, you would have a 20 pack-year history. Likewise, if you smoked half a pack per day for 40 years, you still would have a 20 pack-year history.

When you stop smoking (and I trust you will), note why you quit. For instance, you may have adopted a healthier lifestyle. You also may have been scared by a notable decline in your breathing ability. This can also help your physician understand the whole picture. When you stopped, did you quit cold turkey or use smoking cessation aids or other means to help you stop? How many times did you "quit" before you kicked the habit? How many years ago did you quit? It is never too late. Although you may not be able to reverse the damage already done, you can decrease its progression by quitting.

Aside from cigarettes, do not forget to record the use of other tobacco products. If you never smoked cigarettes but smoked cigars, document the average number smoked each day. Similarly, if you never smoked any form of tobacco but you chew tobacco, specify the number of canisters you usually empty in a week. While smoking cigars and chewing tobacco do not carry all the risks of cigarette smoking, they are also associated with certain risks. Do not omit them from your history.

Your *alcohol history* is also of paramount importance. Excessive alcohol intake has been associated with various types of cancer, including cancer of the breast and esophagus, life-threatening heart, liver, and pancreas diseases, brain shrinkage, and other medical conditions. Many people who drink enough to put them at risk for these potentially serious conditions do not even realize they are in danger. What many call social drinking will rob them of many quality years of life.

When recording alcohol intake, be as precise as you can be. And do not forget to include beer consumption. Beer is an alcoholic beverage. Yet many patients who drink large quantities of beer often answer "no" when asked if they drink alcohol because they associate the word *alcohol* only with hard liquor.

Note how many drinks you consume each week on average. Knowing your approximate history of alcohol consumption may push your physician to consider diagnoses he otherwise might not have. Do not be ashamed to tell the truth. Chances are that if you feel embarrassed, you may be drinking too much, and you might need help so you do not end up with a life-threatening alcohol-related illness one day. Your doctor is not there to judge you. He is there to help you live as long and healthy as possible. If you are not honest about your alcohol consumption, you may pass up an opportunity for confidential help that could save your life.

Occupational exposures can be significant as well. For instance, if you work in a plant with harmful dust and chemical fumes, find out the names of these substances. Likewise, even unobtrusive situations should be well documented because certain occupations carry inherent risks. For instance, food handlers and machine operators have a particularly high risk of contact dermatitis, a skin condition that results from contact between the skin and a substance that irritates it.

Keep a detailed history of not only your job title but also your job description. Be specific about your tasks. Leave nothing open to interpretation. For example, in one company, clerks may spend their days in a plush office entering data into computers. In another, they transfer 75-pound boxes to a warehouse filled with chemical fumes.

In the first situation, the clerk may be at high risk for carpal tunnel syndrome due to repetitive movement of his wrists. In the second case, he may develop a severe back injury from heavy lifting. Alternatively, he may develop lung disease from sniffing dangerous fumes.

Try hard to be as specific as you can be. Even try to list previous jobs and specifics of what you did. Occupational exposures have been associated with various diseases of multiple different organs. Unfortunately, the diagnosis is often missed because there may not have been much training about such vulnerabilities in medical school.

Occupational diseases frequently go undiagnosed because the patient and physician lack understanding. Keep detailed records of your work history. You will increase the odds it will be correctly diagnosed if you ever develop an illness related to your job. However, remember to be concise. Do not write page after page of every little detail of your last 10 jobs. Instead, note specific information on the chart provided in this book. As with other charts in this book, you can download as many blank copies as you like. Use the backside to document details you cannot document in the limited space provided on the front of the chart.

Knowing other potential environmental exposures can also give your physician clues about an illness. For example, let's say your doctor knows every fall, you and "the fellas" go on a camping trip in an area known to have a high incidence of Lyme disease. She may consider this disease a possible cause of some vague symptoms you have. There are special tests to confirm the diagnosis, but if she does not know you are at risk, she may not see a need to order them.

Activities you commonly do in your leisure time should also be included in your social history. Even pet exposures should be included in your account. See the accompanying chart for vital information to include in your social history.

Your doctor may also ask you about current or prior illicit drug use. He may inquire about sexual matters as well. While you may not feel comfortable recording this information in a table, be aware those questions may arise.

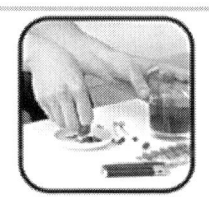

social history

Alcohol Use

Amount Consumed:	Beer	Wine	Hard Liquor
Ounces/day			
Days/week			
# Years			

Tobacco Use

Type:	Daily Amount	# Years Used	Year You Quit
Cigarettes			
Cigars			
Chewing Tobacco			

Occupational Exposures

Hazardous Exposure/Activity	Your Job	# Years

Hobbies

Immunizations/Health Screenings

Each year, countless people die from diseases that are preventable or treatable. Many advances have been made in the medical field. Some conditions once uniformly fatal have been transformed into treatable chronic conditions. Others are completely eradicated. Yet, there is still a long way to go. Keeping up with nationally recommended preventive medicine screening tests can not only save your life but give you a better quality of life. Periodically, recommendations change, but your doctor is an excellent source for updates. The adage, an ounce of prevention is worth a pound of cure, is still alive and well today! In addition, early detection can lead to a complete cure for some previously incurable cancers.

immunizations

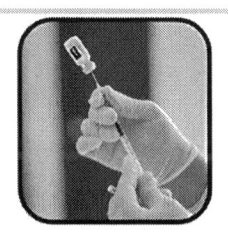

Immunizations	Date	Date	Date
Chickenpox			
COVID-19			
Diphtheria			
Flu (influenza)			
Hepatitis A			
Hepatitis B			
HPV			
Measles			
Meningococcal			
Mumps			
Pertussis			
Pneumococcal			
Rubella			
Shingles			
Tetanus			

List any additional vaccines taken (such as for travel).

Note, the number of boxes doesn't reflect the number of doses recommended.

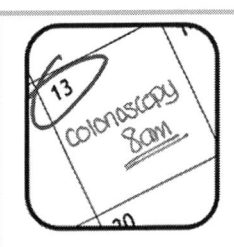

health screenings

Screening	Date	Date	Date
Abdominal aortic aneurysm (one-time)			
Blood pressure			
Cholesterol			
Diabetes			
Breast cancer			
Cervical cancer			
Colorectal cancer			
Lung cancer			
Prostate cancer			

List any abnormal results and follow-up needed.

DID YOU KNOW?

You can pick up a home blood pressure monitor at your local pharmacy inexpensively and help your doctor improve your blood pressure control. Take a log of your readings with you to appointments. Also take your monitor. Check your blood pressure reading against the reading obtained with a professional device regularly to make sure your readings are accurate.

Health Logs

Some chronic conditions are common and significantly increase your risk of developing potentially catastrophic illnesses, such as a heart attack or stroke. High blood pressure, diabetes, and high cholesterol are particularly important. Keep track of your numbers so you can play a more active role in helping your doctor help you. Know your numbers!

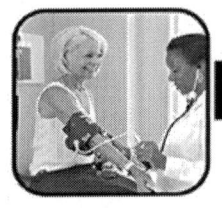

blood pressure log

Date	Time	Blood Pressure	Date	Time	Blood Pressure

BLOOD PRESSURE CATEGORIES

Category of Blood Pressure	Systolic Blood Pressure (upper number)		Diastolic Blood Pressure
Normal	119 or lower	and	79 or lower
Elevated	120 - 129	and	79 or lower
Stage 1 Hypertension	130 - 139	or	80 - 89
Stage 2 Hypertension	140 or higher	or	90 or higher
Hypertensive Crisis *Seek medical attention immediately!*	181 or higher	and/or	121 or higher

REFERENCE: THE AMERICAN HEART ASSOCIATION

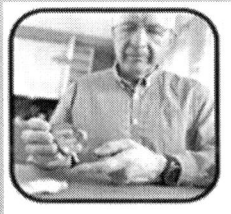

blood sugar log

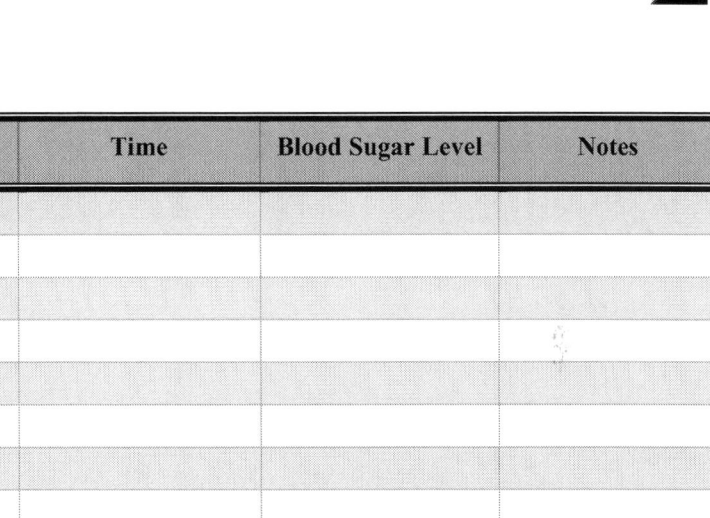

Date	Time	Blood Sugar Level	Notes

Highest reading/extenuating circumstances:

Lowest reading/extenuating circumstances:

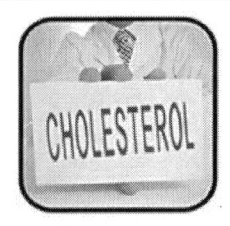

cholesterol levels

Date				
Total Cholesterol				
LDL Cholesterol				
HDL Cholesterol				
Triglyceride Level				
Non-HDL Cholesterol				
VLDL Cholesterol				

Date				
Total Cholesterol				
LDL Cholesterol				
HDL Cholesterol				
Triglyceride Level				
Non-HDL Cholesterol				
VLDL Cholesterol				

Standard lipid panels include total, LDL, and HDL cholesterol levels, as well as triglyceride levels. Some lab reports also include non-HDL and/or VLDL cholesterol levels. But your doctor can extrapolate meaningful information about your risk of clogged arteries from the first four.

Healthy Living Goals

There is more to consider than controlling diseases once you get them. Think about what things you can do to prevent them. A healthy lifestyle goes a tremendous way in decreasing your risk of several common and potentially dangerous medical problems. Set your goals and then work toward them. Your doctor can help you tailor goals that are safe and effective. Following are charts to get your started.

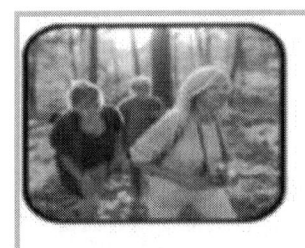

exercise log

Date	Type of Activity	Duration	Notes

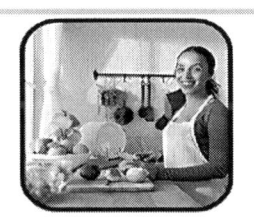

healthy diet log

Date	Servings of Fruit	Servings of Vegetables	Servings of Grains	Servings of Protein	Servings of Dairy

Visit https://www.myplate.gov/myplate-plan to get a sample personalized food plan, based on your sex, age, height, weight, and physical activity. Note, your doctor, not an online guide, can best guide your dietary recommendations based on any chronic conditions you may have and other personal factors.

> *A great way to empower yourself is to invest in your health and eat well by choosing foods packed with nutrients like fruits, vegetables, whole grains, healthy fats, and lean proteins. Eating well isn't depriving yourself - it's getting nutritional bang for buck from most of what you eat. You can still enjoy a treat here and there and thrive!*
>
> **-Jessica Collet Murphy, MBA, MS, RD, LD, CHC**
> **Healthcare Member Experience Analyst**

Correspondence

This section of your personal health record should contain important correspondence, such as a letter written to you by your physician or an insurance statement. In addition, jot down any calls, emails, or letters received for quick reference.

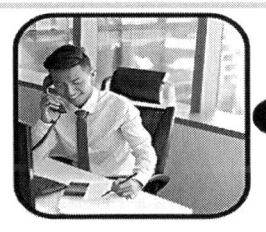

correspondence

Date	Doctor	Reason	Outcome

Test Results

Although you may want to jot down some easy-to-remember test results, such as a total cholesterol level of 150, other tests are too complicated for the layperson to understand fully. The following is part of a sample basic metabolic profile.

	Result	*Reference Range*
Sodium	*143*	*(135-145) mmol/L*
Potassium	*4.0*	*(3.5-5.0) mmol /L*
Urea Nitrogen	*8*	*(6-20) mg/dL*
Glucose	*100*	*(65-120) mg/dL*
Creatinine	*1.0*	*(0.7-1.5) mg/dL*
Carbon Dioxide	*29*	*(24-32) mmol/L*

As you can see, these test results are best photocopied. By keeping copies of your X-ray reports, electrocardiograms (EKGs), and other diagnostic test reports, you can provide a more detailed picture to future health professionals on the spot without having to wait for your old records to arrive. This will help the doctor focus on potential problem areas faster, which can easily translate into a speedier diagnosis with fewer required tests. This will save you time and money and prevent an avoidable delay in your diagnosis and, thus, your treatment.

Advance Care Planning

Insert all pertinent documents pertaining to your health care wishes should you be unable to communicate them in this section. For instance, if you suffer a severe heart attack and could be kept alive only by a ventilator, would you be amenable to this? If there was little hope for meaningful recovery, you might opt not to be placed on it. However, in such a situation, you could not communicate those wishes. All advanced care planning documents should be kept together.

These include:
- Advanced directives
- Living will
- Medical Power of Attorney
- Organ and tissue donation documents
- Do Not Resuscitate or Intubate orders
- Medical Orders for Life-Sustaining Treatment (MOLST), also known as Physician Orders for Life-Sustaining Treatment (POLST), based on which state you live in

Miscellaneous Information

As in most cases, there are issues that will not fit snuggly into a specific category. The last tab in your medical record binder can be a section for miscellaneous information.

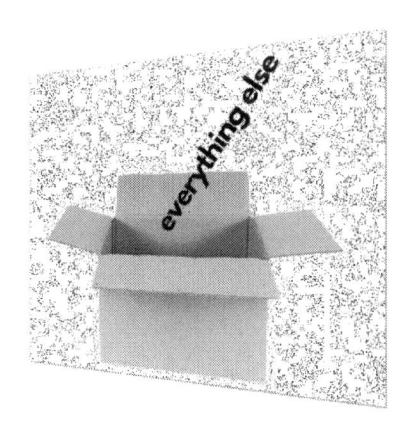

After you have constructed your medical record, study it! Suppose you are in an automobile accident or any other unpredictable situation and find yourself in an emergency room. There, you will not have your record. However, being able to relay the crucial information your medical history contains to your physicians and nurses is as good as having it handy. And always keep a copy of your mini-medical record updated and in your wallet.

The information in this chapter laid the foundation for developing your personal copy of important medical records. Sometimes, you may need more or less extensive documentation. Still, you now have the basic building blocks which will start you on your way to a better-informed, more prepared medical future.

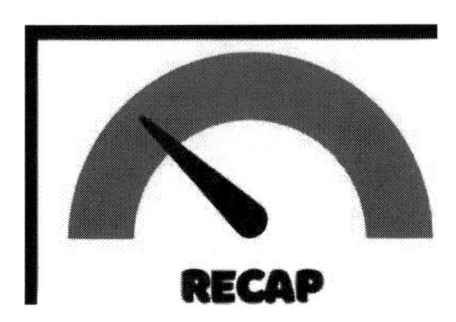

RECAP

- Having a personal copy of your medical records can help expedite your diagnosis.
- It is easy to develop a concise, organized copy of personal health records that is easy to navigate.
- A 3-ring binder with tabs is a simple solution for keeping vital records.
- After you put together your record, study it so you will know the most important aspects of your health history.
- ALWAYS keep a copy of your mini medical records in your wallet.

QUIZ

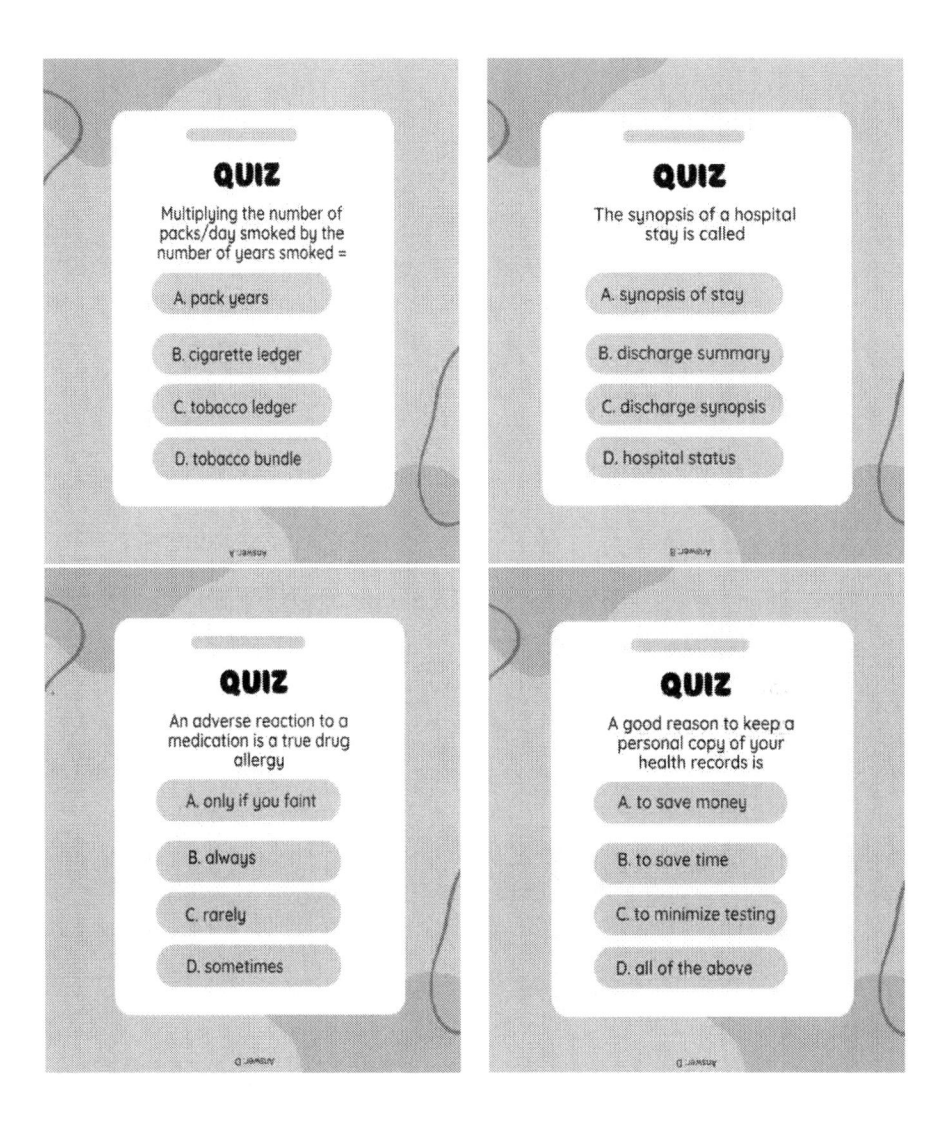

QUIZ
Multiplying the number of packs/day smoked by the number of years smoked =

- A. pack years
- B. cigarette ledger
- C. tobacco ledger
- D. tobacco bundle

Answer: A

QUIZ
The synopsis of a hospital stay is called

- A. synopsis of stay
- B. discharge summary
- C. discharge synopsis
- D. hospital status

Answer: B

QUIZ
An adverse reaction to a medication is a true drug allergy

- A. only if you faint
- B. always
- C. rarely
- D. sometimes

Answer: D

QUIZ
A good reason to keep a personal copy of your health records is

- A. to save money
- B. to save time
- C. to minimize testing
- D. all of the above

Answer: D

Chapter 6

STAY SAFE IN THE HOSPITAL

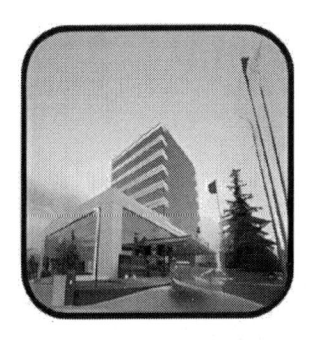

Most of us find ourselves unexpectedly in the emergency room (also known as emergency department) at least a few times. Relax. Not every ER visit ends up in hospitalization. If your condition is not severe, you might not need to stay. For instance, if you have mild dehydration after two days of diarrhea, you may perk up quickly after a bag of IV fluids.

If there is no evidence of anything serious, the ER doctor may discharge you home in a few hours. The next step in your care is to make an appointment to follow up with your regular physician as an *outpatient*. Outpatient care is when you receive medical treatment without being admitted to the hospital.

During this visit, your doctor will re-evaluate your condition to ensure you are improving as would be expected. You may be tempted to forego that visit, especially if you feel 100% better. At the very least, call your doctor to discuss the need for a follow-up visit after a trip to the emergency room. Keep your ER discharge paperwork and show it to your doctor at your next visit. Also, make sure your doctor gets a copy of the emergency room records. He may have computer access to your ER records. If not, he knows the steps to take to get a physical copy of them.

You never know when an emergency may occur. So, have a sense of urgency about having access to your personal health records. If paramedics are called because you have an emergency at work, you want access to your vital health records. The emergency room doctor will want to know specific information, such as your medications and dosages, medication allergies, and prior diagnoses.

There are several options for ensuring ready access to your medical records. For instance, many medical groups and health insurance companies give their patients access to an online health portal. This empowers you to view essential documents about your health on demand.

But if you are too sick to log in, forget your login information, or lack a smartphone or tablet, you may not be able to take advantage of this safety net. This is when having a miniature medical record in your wallet comes in handy. This does not have to be an extensive record of every office visit and procedure you have had in the past 20 years. Instead, focus on the big picture. You can download a copy of My Mini Medical Record from: **http://www.patientempowerment101.com/my-records**. If you need extra room, simply turn the page over and print another copy on the backside of the page. You should keep this updated and stored in your wallet in case of an emergency.

Components of a mini-medical record:
- Your name and number
- Your physician's name and number
- Your pharmacy name and number
- An emergency contact name and number
- Chronic medical conditions
- Medications, including dosages and how often you take them
- Medication allergies/intolerances
- Major surgeries

Medications

If the ER doctor does not know your medications, he is left in the dark about making important decisions. For example, he might not order a drug you need. Or he might order a medication that interacts negatively with medication still in your system. Therefore, knowing your medications is crucial!

When you plan a trip to the hospital (or the doctor), ensure you can quickly give medical providers an updated list of your medications. Either take a bag of all your prescription medications, vitamins, and nutritional supplements or a detailed list of them. Include the name, dosage, frequency, and why you take each. If it is a prescription medication, jot down the prescribing doctor's name.

There are pros and cons to each option. If you take a bag of all your medications and supplements with you, the medical professionals caring for you can count the number of pills you have left in each bottle. Naturally, they will only do this for medications of importance. This can be helpful if you forget to take several doses. It is not uncommon that a person winds up in the emergency room for this reason alone, skipping medication doses.

For instance, if a person has a weak heart, her body may desperately need diuretic medication (fluid pills) to remove excess fluid from her body. Without it, fluid can build up in her lungs, making her feel short of breath. The doctor who admits her to the hospital will want to know what worsened her previously stable condition. If he knows she missed several doses of her diuretic, he may need to look no further for the cause, especially if the lab results are unremarkable.

Everyone forgets things. If you forgot to take a few doses of medication, you might not remember you forgot. That's the nature of forgetting. It's part of being human. You could honestly answer "yes" when asked if you take your medications as prescribed. However, you may be oblivious to the fact that you did miss a few doses. Having a bag with your pill bottles helps doctors reconcile what you remember doing with what you actually did.

Likewise, if you have missed multiple doses of your blood pressure medicine, you would expect your blood pressure to be high. Suppose you are discharged home from the ER. The doctor is less likely to increase your blood pressure medication on discharge if he attributes the high readings to your missing doses. Otherwise, he may tell you to double up on your prescription, thinking it will improve your blood pressure control. However, if your blood pressure was simply high because you had not been taking your medication as prescribed, and you go home and double the dose, your blood pressure may plummet. This could be catastrophic.

The con of bringing in a bag filled with your pills is that you may not have the time to gather the bottles together in an emergency. If you keep an updated list of all your medications, supplements, and vitamins in your wallet, just pull it out in a crisis. But this option decreases the ability to assess how many doses you missed, if any.

To get the benefit of both methods, do both things. Keep a detailed medication list in your wallet. Also, keep your medications and supplements in a central place so you can quickly transfer them all to a bag if you are in a rush. It helps to keep a large plastic zip bag nearby, so you don't have to search for one when you need it quickly. Make sure your spouse, another family member or significant other has quick access to your medication list. Also, if you are a caregiver or have one, ensure you both have a copy of your medications. Every time you update your list, give someone you trust a copy and jot down the date updated at the top.

A mobile app on your smartphone is another viable option for keeping track of your medications. Various medical record-keeping apps help you keep up with your medications and other essential health records as well. Before you download a mobile app:
1. Research it.
2. Read its reviews.
3. Learn about its security.
4. Even ask your doctor for a recommendation.

Don't go alone

If you have a true emergency, like a heart attack or stroke symptoms, call 911 and don't drive yourself to the emergency room! The last thing you want is to risk having a wreck if your condition deteriorates on the way. You could also end up in a traffic jam, a potential nightmare situation unless you're in an ambulance. In a genuine emergency, minutes matter.

If you plan to drive to the emergency room in a less urgent situation, ask a friend or family member to go with you. It's always good to have someone you trust by your side. Understanding medical explanations and instructions can be difficult on a good day. When you are sick, this task becomes even more daunting. Having an extra set of eyes and ears can have tremendous implications. This is especially true if you have problems remembering things. You may forget something important, particularly if given strong pain medication. In addition, your companion may think of questions to ask that you may not think of. She may also help fill in the blanks for the doctor if you cannot communicate effectively for whatever reason.

> *The ED physician is tasked with determining the worst possible thing that may be causing your symptoms and attempting to ensure there is not a life-threatening condition present. It is important to try and be concise in your discussion of what your symptoms are, and it is important to let them know why you came in that particular day and what you are most worried about. You are the center of the care team's focus; you are exactly why they are there caring for you. Please play an active role in the process. Make sure your questions are answered and that you have a clear understanding of what your next steps are, especially if you are being discharged home. Be sure to ask any outstanding questions you have of your care team. There is frequently additional consultation and testing that needs to happen after an ED visit that should be outlined in your discharge instructions.*
>
> *-Chirag Chaudhari, M.D.,*
> *Emergency Room Physician*

Family Matters

Contact a close family member if you drive to the emergency room and no one else is available to go with you. He can notify other people you want him to reach. Also, tell the nurse or doctor the name(s) of individuals they can discuss your condition with when they call to check on you. The Health Insurance Portability and Accountability Act (HIPAA) restricts the ability of medical providers to discuss your private medical information. Violating HIPAA rules can get a medical provider fired. The most egregious cases could even result in jail time!

A ***medical power of attorney (POA)*** document is desirable. This is a directive that lets you appoint an individual to make important health care decisions on your behalf if you cannot. If you do not yet have a POA, make your wishes known. You can ask your doctor to call a specific family member daily and update him on your condition. Appoint one family representative as the doctor is unlikely to have the time to contact multiple family members for updates. This is one way you give your permission to speak with a family member.

If you have several doctors on your case, the family communication is best accomplished by the doctor overseeing your case. He contacts the consultants on your behalf. He will know their plans and their impressions. The doctor who oversees your care is called the ***attending physician***. This is the doctor who officially admits you to the hospital, does daily hospital rounds, coordinates your care, and discharges you. This is also the doctor who prepares your discharge summary with the important aspects of your hospitalization. If he is in a group, one of his partners may take over your care on weekends or at the end of his scheduled time on the hospital wards. Many hospital specialists (***hospitalists***) work 7 days on, 7 days off.

<u>What to take to the hospital</u>
- Your medical insurance card
- Your medication list/bag of medications and supplements
- Cell phone and charger

- Books/magazines
- Tablet or small games you enjoy, such as a deck of cards

> *In addition to all of your medications, medical history, clothes, iPad, and other necessary items, please pack your patience if you are headed to the Emergency Department! It is oftentimes very frustrating for patients and family to sit in the waiting area for hours, without receiving any attention. What they might not realize is that there is a complex, well-developed triage process being utilized to prioritize patients. There is an objective set of guidelines that have been formulated in order to try to take care of patients as efficiently as possible, while also preventing unsafe situations where the sickest patients' needs are addressed first. Although every patient in the Emergency Room feels that their personal situation is the most urgent, in reality, patients and family members would be better served if they understood that we, as ED providers and staff, all want to see and take care of those in the waiting room as quickly as possible. It may feel like you or your family member keeps getting "bumped" for other patients walking in the door. I would ask that you reframe your mindset, and try to reassure yourself or your loved one that this means their situation is more dire than yours.*
>
> **-Sharon Nath, Emergency Room PA-C**

If you are like many people, you haven't memorized the phone numbers of all the essential people in your life. You have a contact list on your cell phone, which lets you call them on demand. But if your battery dies, you might be unable to contact them when you need to if a serious situation occurs. Don't assume that the hospital will have an extra charger that fits your cell phone. Sharing chargers can spread germs, potentially dangerous germs. Always be prepared.

When you go to the ER

If you are admitted to the hospital, you might want somebody to pick up your car. This is particularly true if it's clear that you will not be able to drive yourself home. Ask a family member to bring books or magazines for you to read if you didn't have time to grab any on the way to the hospital. This can be a stressful time. Find activities you enjoy that can help relieve stress.

You or your family member should notify your primary care physician that you're headed to the hospital. This can be helpful for several reasons. First, he can call the ER doctor and give some pertinent history, such as recent abnormal lab results, concerns about your health, or other vital issues. You might spend several hours in the waiting room before getting back to see the ER doctor. When you see the ER doctor, your doctor's office might be closed for the day. Your doctor may not be reachable, and he may not have ready access to your personal health records if he is. Your doctor's partner may be on call for the group after hours. Chances are that doctor will know little about your medical issues.

> *Don't be afraid. If you don't understand, ask questions. Knowledge is power. Empower yourself.*
>
> **-Tiffany Megary, M.D.**
> **Emergency Room Physician**

Let someone know if your condition worsens while in the waiting room. Whenever your health is on the line, speak up. A nurse might need to reassess you. If there has been a significant change, such as a major change in your vital signs, it will expedite your move to an ER room.

Note the name badge of everyone who takes care of you. Expect to see registered nurses, possibly a pharmacist, and an ER provider, such as a physician or physician assistant. The medical professional taking care of you may be an MD (medical doctor), DO (doctor of osteopathic medicine), NP (nurse practitioner), or PA-C (physician assistant).

If you see a non-physician provider, feel uncomfortable, and prefer to see a doctor, you have that right. But realize to be an ER provider, everyone has to demonstrate a high level of competence. They would not be at your bedside if they could not prove this expertise. Likewise, suppose you see a doctor and don't feel comfortable with that doctor because of poor bedside manner or any other reason. There, you can ask to see a different doctor or an Advanced Practice Provider.

Who will take care of you in the hospital?

If you go to the emergency room and need to be hospitalized, the ER doctor will try to contact your doctor. But what if your doctor does not see patients at that hospital or any hospital? In that case, you may be taken care of by a hospitalist. Hospitalists are physicians (or APPs) with expertise in acute, potentially dangerous medical conditions. Their practice is classically limited to hospitalized patients.

Imagine life as a primary care doctor. You may get up early and go to the hospital to see patients before your office opens. Then you turn your attention to your office. You could have a jampacked schedule of patients with others hoping to be fit into another painfully busy day. At 9:30 am, the emergency room calls to tell you one of your patients is in the ER with a stroke. Twenty minutes later, you get a call from a nurse in a hospital ward at another hospital stating that one of your patients is in a downhill spiral and her blood pressure has hit rock bottom due to hemorrhaging from her rectum. Naturally, you can't be in every place at the same time.

It's easy to see why many primary care doctors turn over the care of their patients to inpatient specialists (hospitalists) to divide and conquer. Not to mention it's impossible to keep up with all the major medical advances. For example, a primary care doctor may need to treat a rash between the toes of one patient. The next patient may be feeling depressed because of marital problems. After that, a patient may come in for a routine physical. The variety of patients is vast. Now imagine trying to keep up with all the medical literature for treating toe fungus, depression, disease prevention, and many other conditions. But there's more. He also needs to be on top of information regarding the latest pneumonia that can be rapidly fatal if not treated quickly. And then there's new technology, such as new ways to deliver oxygen to patients whose oxygen level is dangerously low. The list of issues is unending.

Doctors need a work-life balance as well. If married with kids, the demands are even more significant. But that's the beauty of separating primary care from hospital medicine. Some primary care doctors still do go to the hospital. However, others opt to turn over the care of their very sick patients to those who only care for hospitalized patients and keep up with the medical literature to give them the best care. This may be a doctor, a nurse practitioner, or a physician assistant.

Know your hospital status

Do not assume if you are in the hospital, you are formally admitted to the hospital. Your hospital status is essential. There are two major types of hospital status: ***inpatient and observation***. It is vital to understand the difference. The distinction is necessary for insurance reasons, but the care you receive can be the same.

Inpatient status is the traditional status whereby patients who are very sick are cared for in the hospital. Certain conditions typically improve quickly, sometimes within hours, even though the patient looks quite ill on arrival. However, there are other scenarios in which the doctor anticipates a more prolonged and complicated hospital stay, despite receiving excellent treatment. The former would be considered an observation case, while the latter would be an inpatient case. The severity of the illness and the intensity of services required to treat that illness are considered when deciding between observation and admission.

If you are in observation status, you are not then considered sick enough to be admitted to the hospital. Yet, you are too ill to go home. Thus, you are monitored, evaluated further, and treated as needed. After further evaluation, the doctor may find your condition warrants hospital admission. Or he may find you can be safely discharged home to follow up with your private physician.

You may arrive in the ER extremely sick. Let's say you have pneumonia and a low oxygen level. You would rightly expect to be officially admitted from the ER to the hospital with an inpatient status due to the severity of your illness.

But let's say you had severe diarrhea for two days and go to the emergency room due to dehydration. While in the ER, you are considered an *outpatient.* This means you are getting medical care without being admitted to the hospital, like at your doctor's office. Frequently, after evaluation and treatment, ER patients are discharged back home. But suppose the doctor decides you need additional testing and medical care, such as more IV fluids. There, you may be assigned a hospital room. It's important to realize that simply being in a hospital room does not mean an inpatient order has been written. The doctor who takes over your care from the ER physician may anticipate a short hospital stay. You may need a few tests or procedures. For example, you may need one or two more bags of IV fluids. If your clinical condition stabilizes quickly, you might be discharged the following day or even later on the same day. You were observed. You had testing and treatment. You improved rapidly and went home. This is a classic observation case.

A typical observation status symptom is chest pain. You go to the ER one morning due to 30 minutes of chest pain, and the doctor runs an EKG. It does not show a cause for concern, but to be safe, he calls a hospitalist to write orders to send you to a hospital room for further evaluation. At that time, the hospitalist assumes your care. He may order blood tests over time to ensure you did not have a heart attack. By the afternoon, it is clear you did not. Next, he may order a cardiac stress test to look for evidence of blockage of the arteries in the heart that could have caused the pain. The stress test is negative. You go home that evening.

So, you were observed (monitored) while you had further testing to see if there was a serious cause for the chest pain. Your entire hospital stay would be in observation status. But, if the stress test had shown evidence of blood vessel blockage, a cardiologist would typically be consulted, and plans made for a cardiac catheterization. This test allows direct visualization of the arteries of the heart. The stress test showed an abnormality that required more intensive evaluation and management, namely a cardiac catheterization. During this procedure, you may need an intervention to open up the arteries and improve blood flow. In this scenario, your doctor could appropriately write an order to change your hospital status from observation to inpatient.

This delineation between observation and inpatient status is crucial because it can have significant financial consequences. For example, let's say you have Medicare Part A, which covers inpatient admissions but not outpatient or observation services. Unless you also have another insurance, such as Medicare Part B or Medicare Advantage (Part C), you can incur significant hospital expenses while in the observation status. So, it would be best if you always ask about your status. If you have private health insurance, you may receive higher hospital bills when in observation status as well. While observation stays rarely lasted longer than 48 hours in the past, this is no longer the case. So now, you may remain in the hospital in the observation status for several days if warranted. It gets complicated. Don't worry about the details. Let your doctor address that.

Be aware that asking your doctor to order an inpatient admission is not enough. Many health insurers use national guidelines to help determine the appropriate hospital status. Let's take the above scenario when the chest pain was not due to a severe cause. The health insurer would likely deny the bill even if the doctor wrote an order for inpatient status. This could result in the hospital losing a guaranteed payment for observation status in some instances. So, they could receive zero compensation for the care they provided to you. The severity of the illness did not rise to the level requiring an inpatient status based on major nationally recognized guidelines. The bottom line is to know your insurance company's rules for hospital days spent in observation. For instance, you may be surprised to find out that medications given to you are not covered, and you are responsible for paying that portion of your hospital bill. So, ask what your hospital status is and what steps can be taken to minimize your hospital bill safely. For example, your doctor may forego ordering a non-urgent test or two that can be safely done as an outpatient. You never know until you ask.

Tips to optimize your hospital stay

Hand hygiene

Make sure everyone who enters your room washes her hands or uses the hand sanitizer on the wall. This applies to visitors and hospital personnel. There should be no exceptions. Germs can spread rampantly in the hospital. If healthcare providers do not appropriately clean their hands between patients, they can spread potentially serious infections from one patient to another. You also do not want a visitor to bring in any unwanted germs. On the other hand, if your visitors don't wash their hands when they leave your room, they may expose themselves to germs that could harm them.

Medications matter

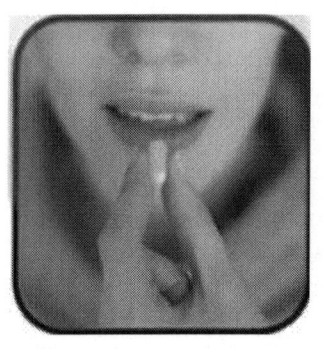

Taking medication as prescribed is an important step toward getting better. If you have even a minor reaction to a medication, ask the nurse to contact your doctor. He may prescribe an alternative medicine. One example is IV potassium. It might cause a burning sensation. If your blood potassium level is very low, you may need your body stores replenished as soon as possible. A low potassium level can not only make you weak and cause muscle cramps, but it can also affect your heart. Some conditions, such as diarrhea and vomiting, can cause your potassium level to drop. If your level is critically low, the doctor might need to give you potassium in your veins and by mouth to increase your levels quickly.

Tell your nurse if you find the potassium in your veins too uncomfortable. Your doctor might ask the pharmacist to dilute the potassium bag with more fluid, decreasing the sensation. This is one of many potential side effects of medications and simple solutions. But if you don't let your feelings be known, the doctor will miss out on the opportunity to keep you as safe as possible, and you could miss out on the opportunity to be taken care of appropriately.

When you get a new medication, ask the name of the drug and why it was prescribed. This will help you understand what you're being treated for and how well each medication helps you. Listen to your body. If you consistently have a headache within 30 minutes of taking a new drug, let the nurse know and discuss it with your doctor.

Hospitals also have a formulary or a list of medications they stock. Don't be surprised if some medications you take at home aren't on its formulary. But there are frequently alternative medications in the same class that can be substituted seamlessly. However, if not or you want to take your own prescription medications, ask if the hospital has a policy to accommodate this request. Many people have family members bring in their medications when it is clear the hospital does not stock theirs. However, never, ever simply take your own medication without notifying the nurse and doctor. This could be disastrous.

If the doctor does not know everything going into your body, he could order a medication that interacts with it in a potentially dangerous way. And the additive effects of too many medications in the same category can be catastrophic. Only after you learn about the hospital policy around taking your own medication should you take anything the nurse does not give you. The policy may be that the pharmacist keeps all medications. You may be given your medication as prescribed (and with the doctor's knowledge), and your pill bottles are returned to you on discharge. The policy may allow you to keep your pill bottles in your room and take them as previously prescribed (again, with your doctor's knowledge). Whatever the case may be, it is imperative that the doctors, nurses, and pharmacists know what you are taking, the dosage, and how often. Even specialists on your case must have clear access to the complete list of medications you are taking in the hospital.

Stay active

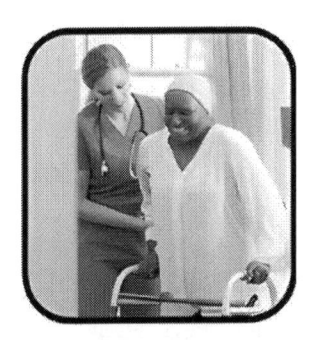

If your doctor has not restricted your activity, get up and move around the room regularly. Make sure you wear no-skid socks or house shoes/shoes when you get out of bed. You don't want to fall on a slippery floor and break a bone. Don't spend all day in bed. The more time you spend in bed, the more your muscles will weaken. This will make it more challenging to return to normal activities when discharged. If your safety is an issue, the physical and occupational therapists might recommend you go to a rehabilitation facility before returning home.

However, suppose you've been walking around regularly throughout your hospital stay. When it's time to be discharged, you are far more likely to be able to return directly home.

Another reason you want to be active is that when you lie in bed for too long, there is an increased risk of developing blood clots. Typically, a blood clot in a leg (***deep venous thrombosis, or DVT***) breaks off and travels through the bloodstream to an artery in a lung, which can be immediately fatal. A blood clot in a lung (***pulmonary embolism, or PE***) can go unnoticed. However, it typically causes shortness of breath and/or chest pain. A warm, swollen, and painful leg may tip the doctor off to the presence of a DVT. A simple ultrasound test can confirm his suspicion. Unfortunately, a fatal PE may be the first sign that a person had a blood clot in his leg. According to the Centers for Disease Control and Prevention (CDC), PE is a leading preventable cause of hospital death.

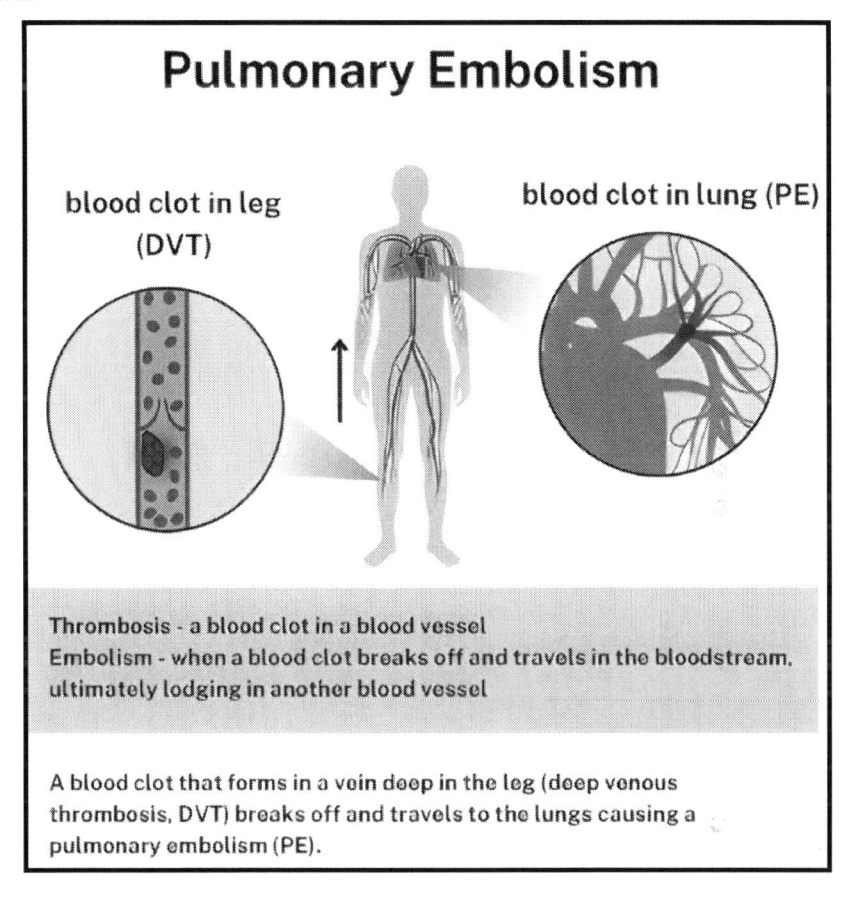

Pulmonary Embolism

blood clot in leg (DVT)

blood clot in lung (PE)

Thrombosis - a blood clot in a blood vessel
Embolism - when a blood clot breaks off and travels in the bloodstream, ultimately lodging in another blood vessel

A blood clot that forms in a vein deep in the leg (deep venous thrombosis, DVT) breaks off and travels to the lungs causing a pulmonary embolism (PE).

Based on your activity level, medical condition, and overall risk of developing a blood clot, your doctor will decide how best to minimize your risk. If he feels you are at low risk, he might just tell you to walk around your room regularly. You're more likely to be prescribed injections if he considers you to be at moderate or high risk for blood clots. Sometimes, your doctor may recommend a mechanical means to decrease blood clots. For instance, there are air-filled devices that go on the lower legs. When they intermittently fill up with air, they squeeze your legs, which increases blood flow. This decreases the risk of blood clots. They are called ***intermittent pneumatic compression devices***.

Talk to your doctor about the best way to decrease your risk of a blood clot. While your hospital might have elaborate checks and balances to ensure each patient gets the appropriate blood clot prevention, systems sometimes fail. Human errors occur. So don't leave it to chance. If your doctor or nurse does not clearly state the plan to minimize your risk of blood clots, ask what needs to be done.

> *Promote your healing and prevent complications such as blood clots and pneumonia by staying active in the hospital. It is easy to feel out of control as a patient, but there are plenty of things you can do to take control of our health and well-being – including staying active.*
>
> **-Dr. Tammy Porter, DNP, MLS, RN, CPHQ, CCM**

Skin breakdown is another consequence of lying around too much. If you or a loved one is too sick to turn over regularly, make sure you are being turned regularly by your nurse or nursing assistant.

DID YOU KNOW?

> *It is vital that you get plenty of rest while in the hospital. Try to maintain your normal sleep-wake cycle, as much as possible. If you are frequently awakened for vital sign checks your doctor may be willing to decrease their frequency. Ask and see. Also, don't nap a lot during the day out of boredom. Open the shades and let the sunlight in. Turn on the room lights and read a book, watch television, or do something else that interests you.*

IV lines

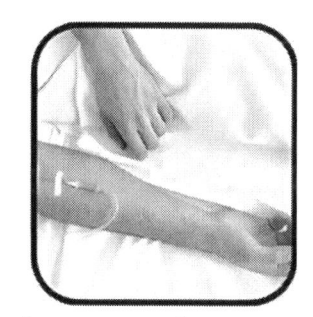

You'll likely have an IV while you're hospitalized. Make sure the site stays clean. An IV catheter site not kept clean might lead to a potentially fatal bloodstream infection. Most often, IVs are placed in a small vein, usually in the arm. IVs placed in a large vein in the neck, chest, or groin area are called *central lines*. Bloodstream infections caused by a central line are called *CLABSIs (central line-associated bloodstream infections).*

While smaller IVs in the arm usually suffice, sometimes you need a larger IV. You may need a central line. There could be several reasons for this. For instance, multiple IVs in the arm may fail to work consistently. You may have veins that are hard to access. Also, if you are in the intensive care unit you may need a central line. Whatever the case, ask your doctor daily on rounds when your central line can be safely removed. Sometimes these large IVs remain in place longer than needed. Your constant reminder may just prompt a speedier, yet safe, removal of this device.

While in place, make sure the bandage covering any IV stays clean and dry. The dressing is a barrier to bacteria, so you want it to function optimally. If you notice the skin near where the IV enters your body is tender, red, or has unusual drainage, notify the nurse or doctor ASAP. It may need to be removed immediately. If you develop fevers or chills while you have a central line, you may need blood cultures to look for evidence of a bloodstream infection, particularly if there is no other obvious source of infection. Finally, avoid touching the IV tubing. Even after washing your hands, they are not considered truly sterile. You don't want to transfer any harmful bacteria to your IV site.

Urinary catheters

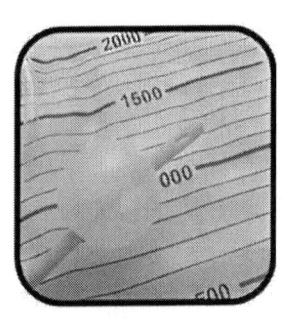

You do not want to have a bladder catheter unless you absolutely need it. Some people prefer the convenience of urinating thru the catheter into a bag without getting out of bed. However, like IVs, urinary catheters can be a path for bacteria to enter the body. *Catheter- associated urinary tract infections (CAUTIs)* are common and potentially dangerous. According to the Centers for Disease Control and Prevention, most urinary tract infections (UTIs) begin in the hospital due to urinary catheters. You may not be aware that sometimes UTIs also lead to bloodstream infections that can be potentially life-threatening. So, get up and go to the bathroom if you are able. If you feel unsteady on your feet, ask for assistance. You can also request a bedside commode and assistance moving from the bed to the commode whenever needed.

CLABSIs and CAUTIs are two of the most significant **healthcare-associated infections (HAIs)**. Each year, tens of thousands of Americans die of a HAI, and their prevention is a top priority for the CDC and countless hospitals across the country.

Consider consults

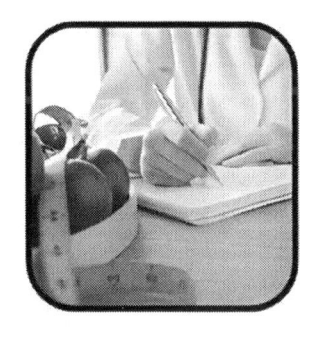

Ask to see a dietitian if you have any dietary concerns, such as how to prepare healthy meals if you have poorly controlled high blood pressure or diabetes. The dietitian could give you invaluable information that can help you control your medical conditions better. Realize, based on how long you are in the hospital and the seriousness of your and other patients' conditions, the hospital dietitian may or may not be able to see you.

If you feel weak, request to see a physical therapist. Note, if you have a well-controlled chronic condition, such as asthma, you will usually not need a consult to see a lung specialist if you are hospitalized for an unrelated reason.

Ask for a business card from all the doctors who care for you, including specialists. They may ask you to see them in follow-up after you are discharged. But remember to check with your insurance company to ensure they are on your plan before making the appointment unless there is an urgent need. Otherwise, your primary care doctor can refer you to another specialist in the same field covered under your insurance plan.

Take notes

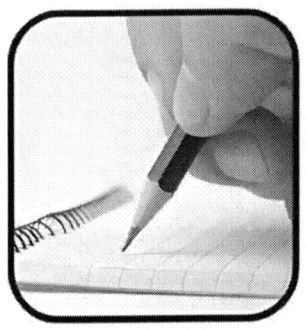

You will likely have multiple blood tests and other diagnostic tests while in the hospital. While you don't need to focus on every negative blood test result, you need to know pertinent positive and negative ones. Let's say you were told your kidneys were not functioning normally due to a medication. The medication was stopped, and the repeat blood kidney test was normal again. You want to know that. If you have access to the hospital's patient portal and can review your test results, do so. You can watch the trends and actual blood test results. Also ask your doctor to review significant test results each day if she does not offer to do so during daily rounds. Don't get caught up in minute details your doctor says are not clinically significant. However, if there's an alert lab value, that may cause concern.

> *Sometimes it may appear that we are not actively intervening. However, healing may be a slow process, and it's then that we treat with what is called "a tincture of time." Always keep a positive attitude. We call it the power of positive thinking. I've seen a lot of crazy things in the hospital, even when things seem hopeless. God works in mysterious ways!*
>
> **- Dr. Raymond Zarate, Hospitalist, Doctor of Nursing Practice**

Get the specific names of all your diagnoses and lab abnormalities. For example, while you might go to the hospital for leg pain, your lab work may show you also have anemia. If it's not severe, your doctor will probably not address it in detail during the hospitalization. However, it is essential to be aware of your anemia because it should be followed up thru your regular doctor.

Prepare for hospital rounds

Ask the nurse the approximate time your doctor does hospital rounds. Having a family member present during daily rounds is beneficial. List questions to ask your doctor each day.

Anticipate hospital discharge

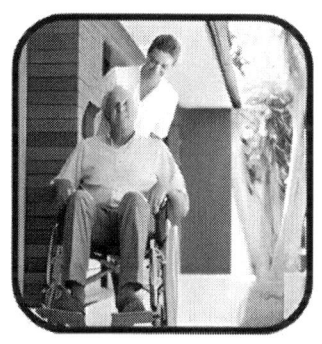

When you are first admitted, ask your doctor how long he thinks you will be hospitalized. That way, you can make your own discharge plans early. While he might not pinpoint the exact day, he might anticipate discharge in two or three days. It may be seven or eight. Either way, when you know the likely duration of your hospital stay, you and your family can plan for your safe transition home and your period of convalescence.

If you cannot be alone after discharge, perhaps someone can take a few days off work to stay with you. Advanced planning makes the day of discharge much smoother for everyone. Sometimes, you may need home medical equipment. If so, ask how and when you will receive it. You may have a case manager who arranges home health issues for you, from home physical therapy to delivering oxygen.

After a medical professional gives you instructions, she may check to ensure you understand them by asking you to repeat the instructions in your own words. If you can do so, she knows she explained things to you in a way you understand. If not, she may need to explain the information differently. It also helps reinforce the instructions in your mind. For instance, at the end of a hospital stay, your nurse may go over your doctor's discharge instructions and then ask you to explain the key points of what she just told you. This is an example of the ***teach-back method***. The ***show-me method*** is another tool a medical professional may use to confirm you understand how to perform a task, such as using an inhaler for wheezing. After being shown how to use an inhaler, you would be asked to demonstrate the technique to confirm you can administer the medication correctly on your own.

Realize there are several potential discharge destinations other than home. Suppose you are weak and need more therapy than can safely be provided at home. There, you may be referred to ***subacute rehab (SAR)***. The rehabilitation will typically occur in a ***skilled nursing facility (SNF)***. An ***acute rehab facility*** may be offered if you need more intensive therapy than you would receive at a SAR. An example is after a stroke. If your condition requires prolonged hospital care, but that care can be provided outside a typical hospital, you may be referred to an ***LTAC (long-term acute care hospital)***. If transferred to an LTAC, anticipate being there for several weeks or longer. An example of someone who may be transferred to an LTAC is someone who has had difficulty getting off a mechanical ventilator. It may take weeks to wean him off the machine successfully. If the other medical issues are stable, this process can occur at this type of specialty hospital.

When approaching discharge, make a list of questions related to discharge. Then, when you see your doctor for the last time, go through the list and ensure you understand the next steps.

Examples include:
- Clarify how you will get any new medications. Also, ask if your medications can be prescribed electronically so they will be ready when you arrive at the pharmacy. If your hospital does not have this capability, ask if it's possible to fax over the prescriptions or call them in (if there are only a few). Have your pharmacy phone number ready. Your final dose of a medication may be scheduled for the evening of your discharge. If your doctor anticipates a late hospital discharge, make sure you can get your prescriptions when needed. For example, if your

medication is called into a pharmacy that closes at seven and you're not discharged until eight, you can miss an important dose. Sometimes, discharges are even delayed until the next day. This results in a prolonged hospital stay and increased costs.
- Ask if any of your medications are expensive and might need prior approval. You don't want to get to the pharmacy only to be told your doctor has to seek prior approval from the insurance company, which can take days.
- Will you get physical copies of your prescriptions?
- When should you see your private doctor for a follow-up visit?
- What warning signs should make you return to the hospital or seek medical attention immediately?
- Do you have any dietary restrictions?
- Are there any physical restrictions?
- Are there any restrictions on driving?
- What new medications will you get and why?
- Does any medication make you sleepy and make it dangerous to drive?
- Should you take your prescriptions, such as nausea medicine, until they're finished, or only if needed?
- When a new prescription runs out, are you finished with that medication, or should you get refills from your private doctor?
- Do you need any follow-up diagnostic tests due to abnormalities found in hospital testing?
- How and when should your doctor expect to get a copy of the discharge summary.
- Are there any pending test results? This is important because an abnormal test result might come back after discharge. If your doctor never received a discharge summary and is unaware of the need to get those results, your health could be at risk. You need to know what tests are still pending, when they'll be ready, and the best way to get the results. If there's a patient portal,

make sure you can access it. Also, make sure your private doctor sees your test results.
- What is the approximate time frame for discharge? You need to make transportation arrangements.
- If you need a return-to-work statement, request it when you see your doctor the last time. Your employer might want any work restrictions or needed time off in writing. Don't wait until you are discharged hours later to ask the nurse. Your return-to-work statement should come from the doctor, and he may have left the hospital before you are officially discharged.
- Ask for handouts explaining your medical conditions so later, you can read up on them.

Finally, the primary doctor caring for you will construct a discharge summary upon discharge. This is a synopsis of your symptoms, physical exam findings, tests and procedures, consultants' opinions, treatments rendered, and other important issues regarding your hospital stay. Technology is imperfect. Sometimes the discharge summary doesn't make it from the hospital to your doctor. The fax machine might malfunction, or the electronic transfer of records might not go thru. It's good to request a copy of your discharge summaries and confirm that your doctor also received her copies. Before your discharge, ask the policy for how you can get a copy of your discharge summary. Although it may not be ready when you walk out the door, the hospital should have a procedure for obtaining a typed copy of the summary when it is available. Keep a copy in your personal medical record file.

> *Never assume that if you don't hear about your test results that it means everything is normal. Always ask your physician when you can expect to hear the results of a test and follow up if you don't receive them in the expected time frame. Labs, hospitals, and physician offices are very busy places and things can and do get missed. However, you need to know if there is an abnormal result that requires follow-up.*
>
> **-Claire Thevenot, MBA, RN, OCN, BCPA, Founder of Clarity Patient Advocates**

As you can see, there are many things to consider when you visit the hospital, whether you are hospitalized or not. Following the recommendations above will make a stressful time potentially much less so. More importantly, they can significantly improve your outcome and safety in the hospital.

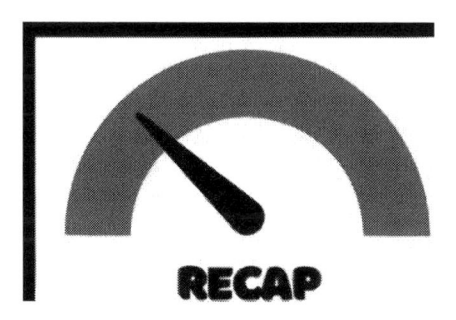

RECAP

- Take your medication bottles with you to the hospital.
- Know your hospital status, observation or inpatient.
- Stay active while in the hospital.
- Get all your questions answered by the doctor before the final visit ends.

QUIZ

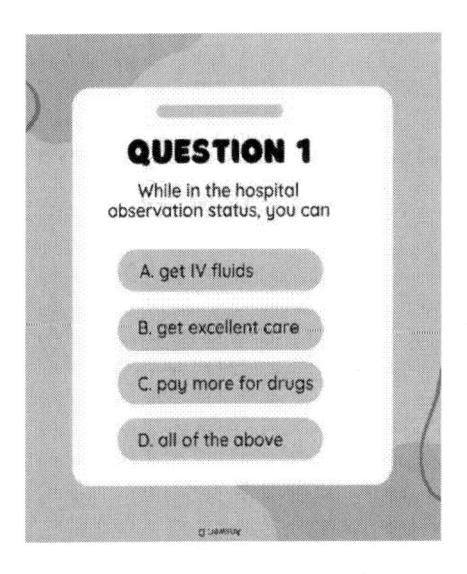

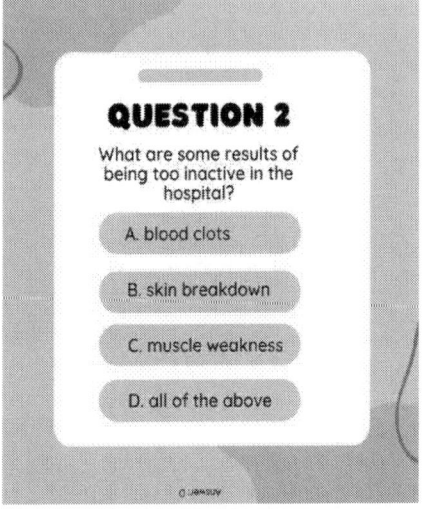

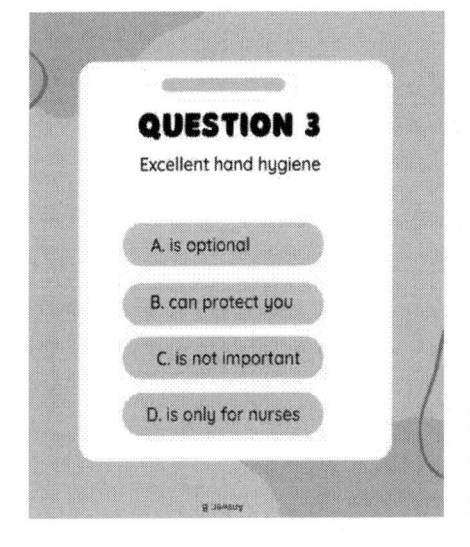

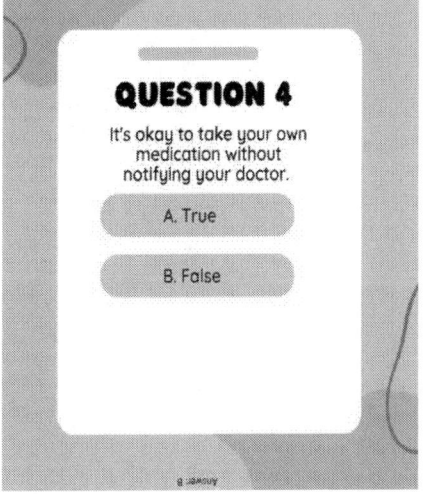

QUESTION 1
While in the hospital observation status, you can

- A. get IV fluids
- B. get excellent care
- C. pay more for drugs
- D. all of the above

Answer: D

QUESTION 2
What are some results of being too inactive in the hospital?

- A. blood clots
- B. skin breakdown
- C. muscle weakness
- D. all of the above

Answer: D

QUESTION 3
Excellent hand hygiene

- A. is optional
- B. can protect you
- C. is not important
- D. is only for nurses

Answer: B

QUESTION 4
It's okay to take your own medication without notifying your doctor.

- A. True
- B. False

Answer: B

Chapter 7

TECHNOLOGY IN HEALTH CARE

Electronic Health Records

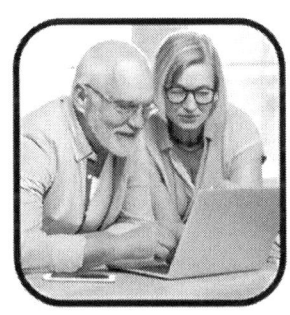

With the widespread adoption of electronic health records (EHR), obtaining old medical records has become much easier, at least for physicians who have adopted this technology. You'll be happy to know these days, the likelihood your doctor uses an EHR is very high. Not utilizing this technology can cost her a great deal of money.

While EHRs date to the 1960s, it was much more recent they picked up steam. A significant reason for this lies in financial incentives. In 2009, the Health Information Technology for Economic Clinical Health Act (HITECH Act) was signed into law during the Obama administration.

This Act rewards "meaningful users" of EHRs thru a federal program. The term "meaningful use" refers to this financial incentive program. Payments are not automatic simply for purchasing an EHR. Eligible healthcare professionals and hospitals who appropriately use EHR technologies to benefit patients and providers must meet specific objectives to participate in the incentive program.

But more importantly, electronic health records are vital and can dramatically expedite much-needed medical care. It was challenging for a physician to get timely access to a patient's old records in the past. For instance, if you went to the emergency room with chest pain, it was once unheard of for the ER physician to visualize your old EKGs within minutes. That is no longer the case. However, the ER physician may still be limited if the place of prior care does not utilize an EHR compatible with the one used by that hospital. Fortunately, some hospital systems have linked EHRs, so a doctor in one city may quickly access records from the care provided in another.

In addition, doctors on call for their partners overnight may also have quick access to records deemed necessary by the treating ER doctor. Some EHRs allow physicians to access medical records securely from a home computer or even a smartphone. Really! So, at 3 a.m., your doctor's partner might log into the laptop on his bedside table and tell the ER doctor treating you what your last EKG showed.

Let's say the ER doctor was contemplating starting a powerful IV blood thinner due to concern about an impending heart attack; the reassurance that your current EKG is unchanged from the one from 3 years ago might quickly change his mind. Since blood thinners can potentially have serious side effects, you want to be spared this exposure unless it is absolutely needed.

High-quality EHRs can help reduce medical errors in many ways. Another example is if there is an error at the pharmacy. The prescription bottle may have incorrect dosing instructions. Suppose you call your doctor to clarify the instructions, and he is unavailable. His nurse can simply check the doctor's note in the EHR and clarify the dosing. This can even take place from another office location.

When healthcare professionals can exchange health information on demand, they are less likely to make medication errors, such as prescribing a medication that is chemically like one that caused an allergic reaction in the past. Even knowing your prior vital signs can be significant. For example, if your blood pressure typically runs low, such as 102/60, a new doctor will not be alarmed if your blood pressure is 100/58 on your first visit. Yet, if she is not aware of what a "normal" day is like for you, she may feel the need to order extra tests and procedures to get to the bottom of what is, to you, normalcy. Many people have relatively low blood pressure with no concerning medical reason.

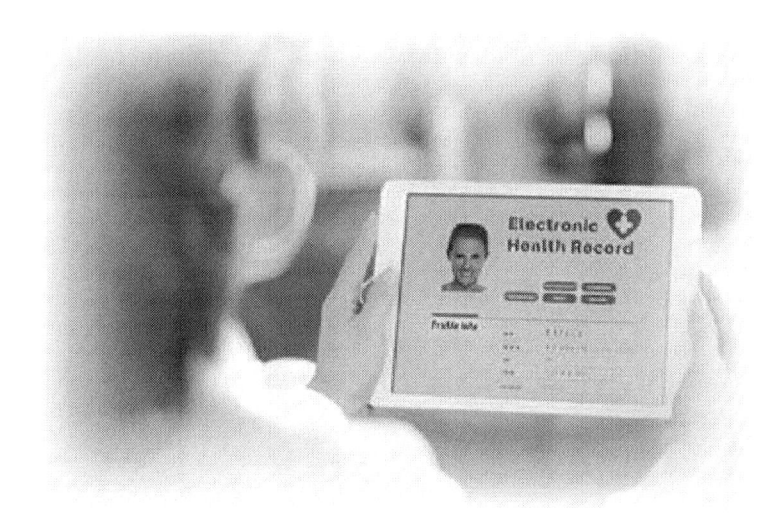

Some EHRs even have a wide range of patient health information that can be printed on demand. For instance, when a patient goes to the emergency room and is diagnosed with a minor illness, such as mild bronchitis, he is typically discharged home. However, a diagnosis as simple as bronchitis may perplex the layperson. What does bronchitis mean? Fortunately, at discharge, it is common for patients to receive printed information that explains the diagnosis in lay terms. This document frequently explains warning signs and when to seek medical attention. Pictures are often included to help patients dive deeper into their health conditions.

From the individual's standpoint, having clear health information is vital. In the past, patients had to rely on handwritten notes from the doctor...if they could read them. Commonly they received no information. Physicians can be extraordinarily busy people. Writing extensive notes for their patients to take home is often unrealistic. Now, they can push a key, and comprehensive literature can be printed out for you. That same information can become a permanent part of your chart. Also, patients can access a wealth of information online regarding their condition when they know what it is called.

Averting medical errors is of tremendous importance. Thousands of Americans die each year because of medical errors. Countless different scenarios can lead to harm. Obviously, health information technology improves healthcare quality by averting medical errors. It also improves communication for both doctors and patients. Boosting efficiency and minimizing waste in the healthcare system are additional bonuses. The utility of this technology is so profound even the federal government places a massive emphasis on it.

Ask your doctor if he has any information to help you understand any topics you feel require further clarification. You can also find high-quality health information online. Unfortunately, some sources are questionable or downright wrong. However, there are multiple reputable sites where a consumer can seek health information.

Due to the COVID-19 pandemic, many aspects of healthcare were ramped up. Learning to complete tasks at breakneck speed and under dire circumstances was a challenge during the pandemic. Technological advances were vital. Due to the high rate of infectivity of the virus, the healthcare landscape had to pivot to a new way of getting things done. One outcome was a surge in telemedicine. Even after deaths due to COVID-19 plummeted, the importance of telehealth visits could not be denied. Whether you live in an apartment in Manhattan or in the wilderness in Wyoming, you can access a doctor on your smartphone, tablet, or computer. These appointments are not meant to replace an ER visit or an in-person visit to the doctor for a potentially serious issue. But they can play a significant role in your healthcare for non-urgent issues.

For instance, if you have an itchy rash on your hand, a quick telehealth visit is an excellent way to get a prescription sent to your pharmacy. Likewise, mild flu, migraines, stomach aches, and multiple other non-urgent conditions can be assessed and treated remotely. Rather than scheduling an appointment, taking off work, driving through rush-hour traffic, then waiting at the doctor's office, you can hop on an appointment online. A telehealth visit is not meant to address a potential emergency; calling 911 is.

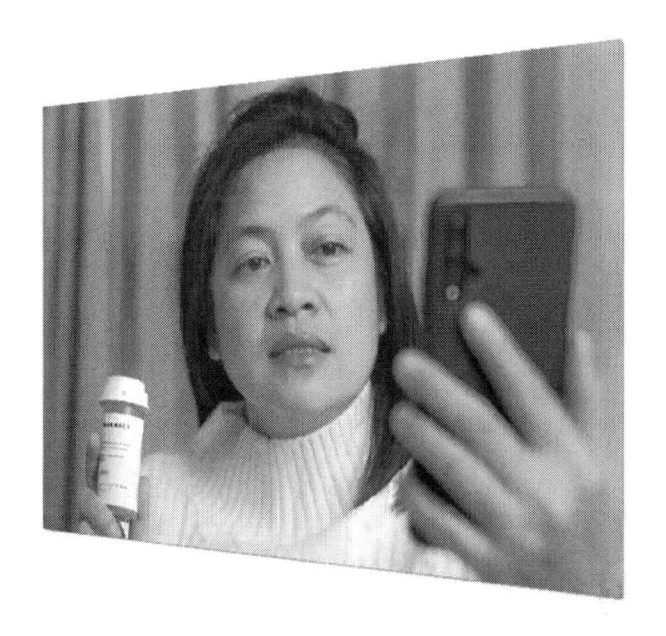

Cutting-edge technology is at your fingertips. Use it. Most people have a smartphone. A simple search on your mobile app store will amaze you. You can keep up with preventive health issues, vaccinations, and much more. You can get medication reminders. You can even find an app that gives an audible alert when it's time to take your medicine. Really! Read the reviews to learn what users say about the app you're considering purchasing. There are thousands of health apps available around the world.

Here are some types of mobile apps you can download today:
- Symptom checker
- Step counter
- Weight loss diet
- Carbohydrate tracker
- Hypertension diet
- Diabetes diet
- Diets for kidney disease
- Monitor heart rate and blood pressure
- Remind you to drink water
- Meditation

- Workout videos
- Sleep tracker
- Healthy habits
- Step counter
- Weight loss
- Prescription saver apps
- Anatomy apps
- Insurance-specific apps
- Breathing exercises
- Sobriety tracker
- Smoking cessation
- Cholesterol management
- Healthy desserts
- Asthma tracker
- Medication reminders
- And many more

But remember, technology, like everything else, has the potential to fail to meet your needs. For example, if your smartphone is lost or stolen, a stranger may access your records. So, when looking for personal health record apps, look for the ones that are most secure and have the means to back up your files. Only you can determine the risk you are willing to take regarding the possibility that your medical records can be accessed by someone who finds or steals your phone. For many people, a stranger learning he has high blood pressure or high cholesterol is not a significant issue. Realistically speaking, a thief will not spend much time trying to learn about your health issues by reviewing an app on your smartphone or looking in the Notes section at your EKG, but again, only you can decide your comfort level.

An app is not a substitute for a physical copy of your personal health records. The portal/server used by the app company may quickly cease to exist if the company shuts down. So, keep a physical copy of your medical records for an emergency.

You can use health information to enhance your life by learning how to adopt a healthier lifestyle. You can also learn how to decrease your risk of significant diseases, such as high blood pressure and diabetes. Why not keep track of national cancer screening guidelines and even learn about the procedures you need to have done to detect cancer early? When you understand what to expect during a test or procedure, you are more likely to go through with it. Fear takes a back seat to knowledge.

Of note, health information can be written on different levels, such as at introductory and more advanced levels. It can also be given in multiple languages, which is crucial.

In addition, you can seek high-quality health information online to help you understand your diagnosis. Some sources are questionable or downright wrong. However, many reputable sites exist where a consumer can seek health information.

There are government sites such as:
- Centers for Disease Control and Prevention (CDC) - https://www.cdc.gov
- MedLine Plus - https://medlineplus.gov

Nationally recognized associations/societies, including:
- American Heart Association - https://www.heart.org
- American Stroke Association - https://www.stroke.org
- American Cancer Society - https://www.cancer.org
- American Diabetes Association - https://diabetes.org
- American Lung Association - https://www.lung.org

You can feel confident in the information you read on government sites and sites sponsored by the above and many other national associations. Evidence-based information is the standard. There are numerous private organizations as well that you can access with a quick Google search using a term such as 'best patient information websites.'

Some examples of highly reputable sites include:
- WebMD - https://www.webmd.com
- Drugs.com - https://www.drugs.com

Note that this is an overview and not a comprehensive list of worthy online health resources. Realize everything you read online is not accurate. Check with your physician before beginning a new health practice based on something you read online.

Also, The National Library of Medicine provides an online tutorial to help you evaluate internet health information. The tutorial can be found at: https://medlineplus.gov/webeval/webeval.html.

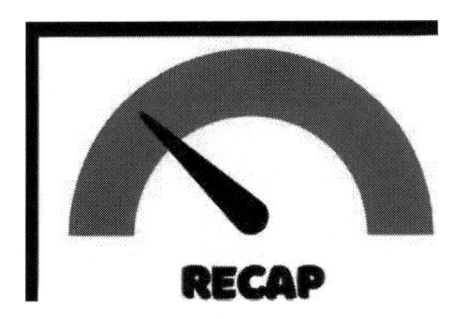

RECAP

- Technology in healthcare is making life safer and more convenient in many ways.
- Telehealth visits can save you a lot of time but schedule them wisely.
- When obtaining health information from an online site, ensure it is reputable.

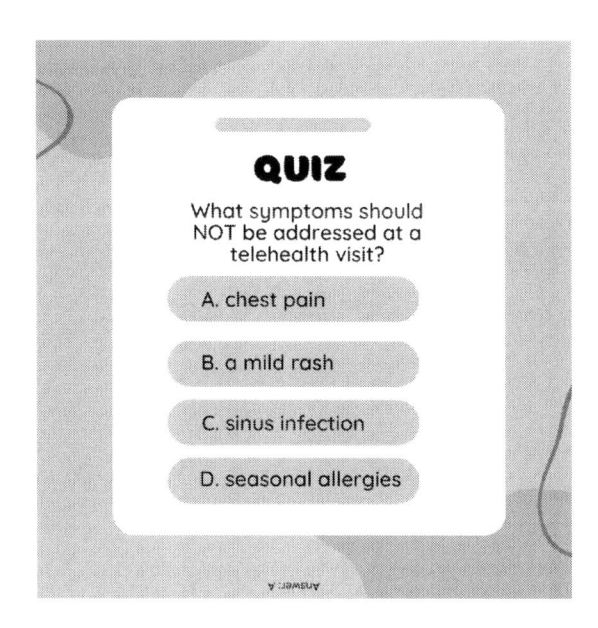

QUIZ

What symptoms should NOT be addressed at a telehealth visit?

A. chest pain

B. a mild rash

C. sinus infection

D. seasonal allergies

Answer: A

Chapter 8

THE POWER OF AN ADVOCATE

Picture this, you've been saving up for a camping trip near the rim of the Grand Canyon for over a year. You rent a luxury RV and invest in all the latest camping technology to make your 2-week adventure the vacation you've always dreamed of. Your food pantry is stocked to the hilt. When the long-awaited day finally arrives, you hop out of bed long before the alarm sounds. After hurriedly getting dressed, you scarf down a quick breakfast, rush to the RV, and take off. You feel a deep sense of contentment as you take in the beautiful scenery 6 hours into the drive. Suddenly, you feel a jolt. Then the RV shakes. Oh no! A front tire just blew out. Luckily, you see a rest station nearby, so you pull over. In your anguish, you glance to your left and see a charter bus for a college football team parked next to you. Several strong young men get out to offer assistance.

Do you:
   a. Take them up on their offer to help you change the tire, or
   b. Thank them for their offer, but reassure them that despite your small stature, you can change the tire on the monstrosity of a vehicle in front of you?

I hope you'll choose 'a' without much thought. Now, picture this, you become ill. Your doctor tells you some test you can't pronounce confirmed you have some disease you've never heard of. You don't know what to do. Several concerned siblings and friends offer to go with you on your next appointment to get more information so they can help you understand what the doctor says and later research your condition.

They want to be there for you when your doctor tells you what to expect next. Naturally, they want you to get the best treatment possible. Your next-door neighbor is a nurse. She offers to help you navigate thru this scary time as well. You politely decline each offer for assistance.

This scenario plays out repeatedly when people, out of pride, fear, or a desire for privacy, forego assistance from others who want to help them with their healthcare needs. Many prefer to keep medical information a secret, sometimes to their detriment. Trusting your healthcare to another person is difficult, but in some cases, it may benefit you significantly. A spouse, friend, or caregiver can advocate for you. They can function as a second set of eyes and ears regarding health-related issues and speak up if they see anything amiss. Many people could benefit from having a health advocate, but most do not.

Even if you are extremely healthy and exceptionally intelligent, there may come a time when you need someone in your corner. How do you attentively listen to important information from your doctor or nurse when you feel horrible and just want to turn over and close your eyes? Or, while in the hospital you can't seem to get enough sleep because of all the interruptions for lab draws at 5 am and vital sign checks late at night. Are you sure you will understand everything told to you when the doctor sees you at 7 am? Probably not.

It's okay to be a private person. But realize there may be times when you need to loosen your grip on your privacy for your own good. Strongly consider having a medical advocate, whether it is your spouse, significant other, sibling, or someone else you trust. Share vital information about your health so they can help intervene if needed.

If you prefer to keep your medical issues private, consider the services of a professional patient advocate. The role of your patient advocate is to act as a liaison between you and the healthcare providers. You may need help on routine doctor's visits. Or you may go to the hospital seeking care and guidance in a setting that may not make much sense to you.

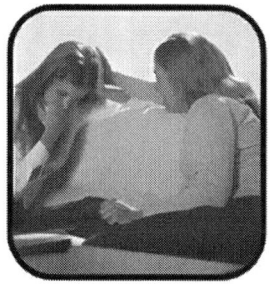

Often, gaps can form between you and your healthcare providers. Your patient advocate is responsible for bringing your concerns to the forefront and ensuring they are heard.

> *People must be active participants in their health and healthcare. When they do this, we all win. Being prepared with advanced directives, an up-to-date list of all your medications and supplements, names and phone numbers of your medical team, links to all your patient portals and current insurance information are important for all to have written down and shared with those who are close to you. Take time to prepare for your doctor's appointment and ask someone to go with you. Prepare questions you want to ask – even for routine visits! If you feel lost or not listened to, consider obtaining the help of a patient advocate.*
>
> **-Anne Llewellyn, MS, BHSA, RN, CCM, CRRN, CMGT-BC, FCM, Founder of NurseAdvocate.com**

Practically, patient advocacy may entail explaining hospital policies while calming you down and relaying hospital information in a way that is easy to understand. Patient education is a significant role played by the advocate. Sometimes medical providers use jargon when referring to hospital terms which can go over your head. Patient advocates can accompany you to appointments, review medical findings, and help you understand your prognosis.

Below are just some of the potential services a patient advocate can provide:
1. Act as a liaison between you and your doctors and insurance company
2. Help you choose medical providers
3. Help you understand your treatment options

4. Explain health policies
5. Schedule and attend medical appointments with you
6. Monitor tests and treatments
7. Support you with complicated insurance paperwork
8. Help with legal documents
9. Arrange meetings with attorneys
10. Assist you in finding support groups
11. Help negotiate medical bills
12. Assist in finding second opinions

Patient advocates can also smooth the transition from inpatient care to outpatient care by explaining medication and how all the outpatient procedures will work. In addition, after you are discharged from the hospital, you may get a long and confusing medical bill. Your patient advocate can break these items down for you and ensure you understand what you're paying for. They can also comment on the correctness of your hospital bill. They might find it easier to pick up on incorrect or double billing than you may. Google "patient advocate near me" and remember to do your research. Ask questions. Compare patient advocates before making a final decision.

Patient advocates are in your corner to relieve any anxieties you may have regarding a new diagnosis, procedure, or treatment. Their job is to break down each situation and ensure that the desired outcome is in your favor. Choosing a patient advocate carefully is essential, especially if going via a private company. It makes sense to include family and close friends in your health decisions so the people closest to you know your medical wishes.

Health advocacy is prominent among the elderly. Advocates can talk to you and determine whether the healthcare being provided is adequate. They may even be able to assist with sourcing food and housing for a patient who may not be able to do so for themselves.

You may choose a ***Medicare Beneficiary Ombudsman*** as well. These professionals can assist in solving disputes and giving you helpful advice. For more information, contact Medicare.
- 1-800-MEDICARE (1-800-633-4277)
- https://www.cms.gov/center/special-topic/ombudsman/medicare-beneficiary-ombudsman-home

Conclusion

I sincerely hope this book helped shed significant light on the complex maze of the U.S. healthcare system. I trust it will empower you to take a previously unimaged step toward optimizing your own medical care. I have enjoyed sharing over 25 years of expertise with you and hope you will help educate those around you about the many tips you learned by reading this book. In closing, I would like to share a quote from an esteemed colleague and dear friend.

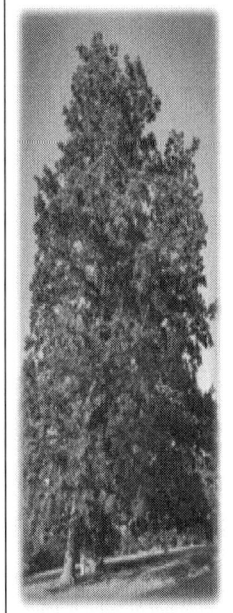

> *As a Nurse practitioner, I have met many families suffering from all stages of grief. I met one memorable family who felt the world's weight was on their shoulders. I was particularly interested in this family because they had weathered many health storms and were here amid another health storm. I reminded this family of what my grandmother always said the morning after a brutal southern storm. I vividly remember after one such storm, my grandmother looked out her window, smiled, and said, "Look at that oak tree; before the storm, it was leaning, and one would have thought it would fall, but it did not. Look at all those other trees on the ground." Like the mighty oak tree, my grandmother said that people endure many storms, trials, and tribulations. Similar to the oak tree, people may lean over, and their sickness may drag them down, but they do not fall; they, too, can survive. My grandmother always said, "it's not the leaning tree that falls."*
>
> <u>*Sometimes it takes patient empowerment to help solidify your foundations.*</u>
>
> -Margaret E. Delgado, DNP, ACNP Board Certified

God bless you,
Your friend, Ann

Appendix 1

Common Medical Tests

This section acquaints you with commonly performed tests. It is not meant to turn you into a medical expert. It should augment your conversations with your physician, not supersede them.

Some of the more common risks are listed for each test, although in most cases, even these more common risks are unlikely. However, in some circumstances, additional risks may be involved, so ask your physician what issues you need to consider before a test. This is not an all-inclusive list. Such a list would be exhaustively long and complicated. The tests listed below are among the more commonly ordered tests, but again, there are many other medical tests a doctor may order based on what he is looking for.

Complete Blood Count (CBC)

Indications: Complete blood counts are frequently performed because they give important information on the status of the different blood cell components. For instance, the white blood cell count is increased with many infections and in certain other conditions. Although it is well known that the count is decreased in advanced HIV disease, a variety of other conditions also classically lower the white blood cell count. Knowing if this cell count is high, low, or normal, the physician can narrow her list of possible diagnoses.

Potential Risks:
To perform a CBC, as with most other blood tests, a blood sample is obtained by puncturing a vein (usually in the arm) with a needle. This procedure is called ***venipuncture.*** Although it is possible for the needle inadvertently to be introduced into a nearby artery, nerve, or tendon,

routine venipuncture is generally a safe procedure. Other than an occasional bruise at the site, complications are uncommon.

Terms your physician may use when discussing results:

- **Anemia** - a low concentration of red blood cells. Once anemia is confirmed, its cause can be sought. Anemia is a common disorder due to conditions as natural as monthly menstrual bleeding or as severe as an acute hemorrhage from as-yet-undiscovered colon cancer. There are numerous causes of anemia, and many individuals are anemic at some point. Not only can a CBC document anemia, but it can also give insight into its cause. There are parameters within a CBC that indicate how large or how small the red blood cells are. Some forms of anemia typically result in small cells, such as iron deficiency. Others cause large cells, such as vitamin B12 deficiency. However, in many cases, the size of the red blood cells in anemic patients is normal. Therefore, knowing the approximate size is valuable to physicians searching for the underlying cause of anemia.
- **Bands** - an immature population of a class of white blood cells. Bands are released into the bloodstream prematurely when the body needs more cells to help fight acute infection. Therefore, their presence in large numbers may signify a potentially serious infection. However, there are other reasons one may see bands as well.
- **Bandemia** - the presence of an excess number of bands in the bloodstream
- **Erythrocytes** - another name for red blood cells
- **Hematocrit** - a measure of the volume of red blood cells in the bloodstream
- **Hemoglobin** - the oxygen-carrying component of red blood cells. The hemoglobin level indicates the concentration of red blood cells in the bloodstream. The ratio of hematocrit to

hemoglobin is typically 3:1. (Hematocrit would be approximately 45 when the hemoglobin is 15.)
- **Leukocytes** - another name for white blood cells (see *white blood cells* below). There are different classes of leukocytes, which include:
  1. polymorphonuclear leukocytes (PMNs)
  2. lymphocytes
  3. monocytes
  4. basophils
  5. eosinophils

  The first three classes comprise the bulk of the circulating white blood cell concentration.
- **Leukocytosis** - an increased number of circulating white blood cells. This is often seen during an infection, although other conditions can cause leukocytosis.
- **Platelets** – particles very important for blood clotting. If they are not functioning well or their number is low, you may bleed excessively from even a minor cut. Platelets are not true cells.
- **Red blood cells** - the blood cells that carry oxygen to cells throughout the body
- **White blood cells** - the blood cells that play a significant role in protecting your body from infection and various other diseases. They are part of your immune system.

Chemistry Profiles

Indications: Blood chemistry/metabolic tests can be basic or more extensive. They are often called a basic metabolic panel (BMP) or a comprehensive metabolic panel (CMP). The former may include 7 or 8 tests, while the latter typically has 14. A BMP focuses on vital blood electrolytes, kidney function, blood sugar, and calcium. Comprehensive profiles add additional tests to the BMP and give a more detailed picture of your overall health. There are numerous chemical substances in the blood. A significant aberration in the concentration of certain ones can be immediately life-threatening. For instance, a very high blood potassium level can lead to cardiac arrest. An abnormal liver enzyme result may result from liver inflammation. Still, it is not acutely dangerous. An example is the elevation of the enzyme alanine aminotransferase (ALT). Elevation is a possible indicator of liver inflammation, possibly due to many causes.

Potential Risks:
This blood test requires routine venipuncture, so the risk is minimal.

Terms your physician may use when discussing test results:

BMP:
- **Sodium** – a major electrolyte
- **Potassium** – a major electrolyte
- **Chloride** – a major electrolyte
- **BUN** (blood urea nitrogen) - an indicator of how well the kidneys are functioning, although, occasionally, the BUN may be elevated in the face of normal kidney function
- **Creatinine** – a stronger indicator of how well the kidneys are functioning
- **Glucose** - blood sugar
- **Bicarbonate** - an indicator of the acid-base balance of the blood
- **Calcium** – a vital mineral in your body

CMP includes the BMP plus additional tests:
- **Alkaline phosphatase** - an enzyme that, when elevated, typically signifies liver or bone abnormalities
- **ALT** – an enzyme marker of liver injury or disease
- **AST** – another enzyme marker of liver injury or disease
- **Total protein** – the measure of essential proteins in the blood
- **Albumin** – a specific protein made by the liver
- **Bilirubin** – a normal waste product of red blood cell breakdown

*Other pertinent terms:
- **Hypercalcemia** - a high blood calcium concentration
- **Hyperkalemia** - a high blood potassium concentration
- **Hypernatremia** - a high blood sodium concentration
- **Hypocalcemia** - a low blood calcium concentration
- **Hypokalemia** - a low blood potassium concentration
- **Hyponatremia** - a low blood sodium concentration

Note that there may be a slight variation in the tests included in the panel based on the laboratory.

Chest X-Ray

Indications: Chest X-rays assess the lungs, heart, and ribs. Physicians frequently order a chest X-ray in patients with a concerning cough, shortness of breath, chest pain, suspected pneumonia, or other conditions. Chest X-rays are good for assessing the anatomy, but not the function, of the heart and lungs; they are also not useful in assessing the details of the heart, such as the arteries and valves.

Potential Risks:
Minimal radiation

Terms your physician may use when discussing results:

- **abscess** - a collection of pus
- **atelectasis** - collapse of a segment of the lung
- **calcification** - deposition of calcium in tissue
- **consolidation** - solidification of a section of the lung, usually due to a pneumonia
- **granuloma-** a noncancerous, usually small, mass that often results from the lungs' reaction to a foreign substance

- **hyperinflation** - overinflation of the lungs often seen with asthma or emphysema
- **pleura** - the paired membranes that line the lungs and inner chest wall
- **pleural effusion** - an abnormal collection of fluid between the pleura
- **pneumonia** - an infection of the lung tissue
- **restrictive lung disease** - one of a class of diseases that prevents the lungs from fully expanding

Thyroid Panel

Indications: The thyroid gland in your neck is a major gland that impacts various bodily functions. It produces very important hormones. When over or underactive, it can cause a wide variety of symptoms. Thyroid panels typically check the level of the 3 major thyroid hormones. Thyroid function tests are performed to monitor known thyroid disease and to screen for evidence of thyroid disease in individuals with signs or symptoms of a thyroid disorder, such as abnormal weight gain or loss.

Potential Risks:
This test requires routine venipuncture.

Terms your physician may use when discussing results:

- **euthyroid state** - normal functioning of the thyroid gland
- **Free T4** – a thyroid hormone
- **Free T3** – a thyroid hormone
- **Total T3** – a thyroid hormone
- **hyperthyroidism** - an overactive thyroid gland
- **hypothyroidism** - an underactive thyroid gland

- **TSH** -thyroid-stimulating hormone. This is a sensitive test of thyroid function that helps determine hyperthyroidism (overactive thyroid) or hypothyroidism (underactive thyroid).

Hemoccult of the Stool

Indications: Testing stool for occult blood (that which cannot be seen with the naked eye) is a common test. This test detects heme, a pigment found in red blood cells. Not infrequently, there is a slow oozing of blood, so not enough is present to notice. There are several potential causes of blood in the stool.

Potential Risks:
There are no significant risks involved in this test since it only entails taking a small portion of a stool sample and smearing it on cardboard slides.

Terms your physician may use when discussing results:

- **heme-negative stools** - the test detected no occult blood in the stool
- **heme-positive stools** - the test detected occult blood in the stool
- **hemorrhoids** - enlarged blood vessels in the anal region

Electrocardiogram (EKG)

Indications: Electrocardiograms give essential information about the electrical activity of the heart. The EKG machine can construct an electrical picture of the heart's activity by placing monitors, called electrodes, at various places on the body. This picture tells a story. For example, the doctor can detect evidence of inadequate blood flow to the heart based on the direction and magnitude of different inflections, called waves. The EKG also gives information about scar tissue in the heart muscle. A scar suggests a prior heart attack. The relative size of the four heart chambers, the origin of the heart's impulses, and other vital information can also be gleaned from an EKG.

EKGs pick up the heart's electrical activity at the chest's surface. **P waves** represent the electrical excitation of the atria that causes them to contract. Likewise, the **QRS complex** represents the activity leading to the ventricle contraction. **T waves** represent the activity of the ventricles as they are relaxing and filling up with blood in anticipation of the next wave of the cardiac cycle. The letters P, Q, R, S, and T denote various phases of the cardiac cycle detected on an EKG.

This set of events happens repeatedly. Electrical impulses are usually generated in the heart's natural pacemaker, the **sinus node.** From there, these impulses pass throughout the heart muscle, resulting in a coordinated series of contractions that pumps blood throughout the body.

When present, a **Q wave** suggests scar tissue in the heart, a finding that points to an old heart attack. Another vital component of the EKG is the **ST segment.** When the ST segment lies above or below the standard baseline, it often signifies decreased blood flow to the heart muscle, as occurs with coronary artery disease. Multiple factors go into a doctor's interpretation of an EKG. This is a general overview.

Potential Risks:
There is a low risk of skin irritation where the leads are placed on the chest wall.

Terms your physician may use when discussing test results:

- **arrhythmia** - an abnormal heart rhythm
- **atrial fibrillation** - a common arrhythmia that starts in the upper chambers of the heart, the atria. It can cause a fast heart rate.
- **AV block** - block in the electrical conduction system between the atria and ventricles
- **first-degree AV block** - a low-level block, often of little clinical significance

- **second-degree AV block** - a more serious block than first-degree AV block:
  o types:
    - **Mobitz type 1**
    - **Mobitz type 2**
- **third-degree AV block** - potentially very ominous. A pacemaker may be required.
- **bradycardia** - a slow heart rate (less than 60 beats per minute)
- **bundle branch block** - a block in a branch of the electrical conduction system of the heart. It may involve the right or left side of the bundle; thus the terms **right bundle branch block** and **left bundle branch block.**
- **dysrhythmia** - another word for arrhythmia
- **infarction** - the death of tissue resulting from severe oxygen deprivation (due to a blocked artery); a myocardial infarction is a heart attack
- **inverted T waves** - upside-down T waves, often indicating ischemia
- **ischemia** - inadequate blood flow, usually due to blockage of the arteries
- **junctional rhythm** - an arrhythmia in which the heart rhythm originates from a site in the junction between the atria and ventricles instead of in the sinus node
- **leads** - a standard EKG consists of 12 leads, or angles, for picking up the electrical activity of the heart
- **left atrial enlargement** - enlargement of the left atrium
- **left ventricular hypertrophy (LVH)** - enlargement of the muscular wall of the left ventricle, often due to hypertension
- **myocardial** - heart muscle
- **Q waves** - an EKG sign of scar tissue, usually signifying a completed/prior heart attack (as opposed to an acute heart attack)
- **right atrial enlargement** - enlargement of the right atrium

- **right ventricular hypertrophy (RVH)** - enlargement of the muscular wall of the right ventricle
- **sinus arrhythmia** - implies that although the heart's rhythm is initiated in the sinus node (as is normal), there is a minor, often insignificant, variation in the frequency of these impulses
- **sinus rhythm** - implies that the heart rhythm is initiated in the normal "pacemaker" of the heart, also known as the sinus node
- **ST depression** - depression of the ST segment, frequently indicating ischemia due to inadequate blood flow
- **strain** - a variation of the ST segment often seen on EKGs in patients who have left ventricular hypertrophy, an enlargement of the muscular wall of the left ventricle
- **ST segment elevation** - elevation of the ST segment frequently indicates myocardial infarction (heart attack), though this is not always the case. Your doctor can clarify this for you should he note this finding.
- **tachycardia** - a fast heart rate applied to rates greater than 100 beats per minute
- **ventricular fibrillation** - a frequently lethal, highly disorganized cardiac rhythm of ventricular origin; one form of cardiac arrest (noted for informational purposes)
- **ventricular tachycardia** - a potentially life-threatening cardiac rhythm in which the impulse originates in ventricular tissue; can lead to cardiac arrest

Holter Monitoring

Indications: Holter monitors are ambulatory EKG recorders. They allow recording the heart's electrical activity over a prolonged time. A lightweight, small recorder is connected to the chest wall by monitoring electrodes, and the patient performs their regular daily activities. Abnormal symptoms, such as lightheadedness or heart racing, can be

recorded in a diary. A few common reasons to perform holter monitoring include:
- To detect abnormal heart rhythms in patients with suspicious symptoms, such as fainting spells or heart racing.
- To evaluate the effect of exercise/activity on heart rhythms
- To assess the impact of medication used to reduce abnormal heart rhythms
- A person has a pacemaker, and there is a concern about malfunction
- As part of the evaluation and management of certain heart conditions.

Potential risks:

You may experience skin irritation where the electrodes attach. Typically, this is not a concern.

Terms your physician may use when discussing test results:

- **atrial fibrillation** - a common arrhythmia that starts in the upper chambers of the heart. It can make the heart rate very fast.
- **atrial flutter** - another arrhythmia that originates in the atria
- **bradycardia** - a slow heart rate (less than 60 beats per minute)
- **dysrhythmia** - another term for arrhythmia, an abnormal heart rhythm
- **junctional rhythm** - an arrhythmia that originates at the junction between the atria and the ventricles
- **premature ventricular contractions (PVCs)** - extra heartbeats that arise in the ventricle
- **supraventricular tachycardia (SVT)** - a very rapid heart initiated *above* the ventricles, thus the term *supra (above) ventricular*.
- **tachycardia** - a fast heart rate (above 100 beats per minute)

Computerized Axial Tomography (CAT scan, AKA CT scan) and Magnetic Resonance Imaging (MRI) scans

Indications: Computed tomography (CT scans, also called CAT scans) and MRI scans are very specialized tests that can be done on any body area. They give detailed images of the internal structures of the body. They are not indicated for all diseases, but they help immensely diagnose and follow numerous conditions. Often, MRIs provide more detail than CT scans. Still, the specific test your doctor orders will depend on your condition. For many conditions, a CT scan or MRI is unnecessary and a waste of money and time.

Potential Risks:
CT scans:
- Radiation exposure
- Allergic reaction to the contrast dye
- With multiple scans, the risk of some cancers may increase

MRI scans:
- Allergic reaction to the dye
- You could be harmed if you undergo an MRI and have metal in your body that is not safe for MRIs. The implications differ based on the metal/device in question.

Terms your physician may use when discussing this test with you:
The terms used will depend upon the area of the body imaged.

Lipid Panel

Indications: A lipid panel is a blood test that measures fat molecules in the bloodstream called lipids. Your lipid levels refer to the types of cholesterol and another type of fat in the blood called triglycerides. High cholesterol increases the risk of heart attacks and strokes. Knowing your numbers is important since steps can be taken to decrease your risk.

Nevertheless, many people who will eventually develop coronary artery disease are not initially considered high risk, so everyone should be screened for high cholesterol.

Potential Risks:
This test simply requires routine venipuncture.

Terms your physician may use when discussing results:

- **HDL cholesterol** - HDL stands for high-density lipoprotein. A high HDL cholesterol level is good to have. It actually affords some protection from coronary artcry disease. It helps counterbalance the bad cholesterol, or LDL cholesterol.
- **LDL cholesterol** - LDL stands for low-density lipoprotein. A high LDL cholesterol level significantly increases the chances of developing blocked arteries, also known as ***atherosclerosis.***
- **Total cholesterol** – Calculated as follows: Total cholesterol = LDL + HDL + 20% (1/5th) of the Triglyceride level.
- **Triglycerides** - a fat related to the food we eat. A high triglyceride level has also been linked to heart disease.
- **VLDL cholesterol** – VLDL stands for very low-density lipoprotein cholesterol. It is typically only present in low amounts in a fasting blood sample. It is from food recently eaten. When increased, it may signify abnormal metabolism of lipids.

Urinalysis (UA)

Indications: A urinalysis (analysis of urine) is usually performed to look for or monitor several conditions, such as a urinary tract infection (UTI), diabetes, liver disease, and kidney disease.

Potential Risks:
There are no significant risks of having a urinalysis because it simply requires collecting a urine specimen in a cup. However, in some

hospitalized patients, a nurse inserts a catheter into the bladder to obtain the urine. Even in these cases, there is a low risk of any problems.

Terms your physician may use when discussing results:

- **acidity (pH)** – measures acidity of the urine
- **bacteria or yeast** – may signify a urinary tract infection
- **bilirubin** – normal product of the breakdown of red blood cells; its presence in urine may be due to liver problems
- **casts** – proteins potentially due to a kidney disorder
- **concentration** – measure of concentration of particles in the urine. Not drinking enough fluids can raise the concentration.
- **crystals** – a potential sign of kidney stones
- **cystitis** - inflammation of the bladder, usually due to a bladder infection
- **glucosuria** - the presence of an abnormal amount of glucose in the urine. While glucosuria is often found in patients with diabetes, it is also occasionally found in healthy individuals without this disease.
- **hematuria** - blood in urine
- **ketones** - a product of metabolism that can be found in the urine under certain circumstances, such as during fasting or with poorly controlled diabetes
- **leukocyte esterase** - a test for white blood cells in the urine; their presence may signify a urinary tract infection
- **nitrites** - another test for white blood cells in the urine; their presence may signify a urinary tract infection
- **proteinuria** - protein in the urine
- **red blood cells** – when found in the urine may signify kidney or other disorder
- **specific gravity** - a measure of the concentration of urine
- **white blood cells** – when found in urine may signify a urinary tract infection

This is a very abbreviated list of medical tests, indications, and results. Ask your doctor why he orders tests for you so you can do your own research, should you so desire.

Appendix 2

Common Medical Abbreviations

1. ABG - arterial blood gas
2. AFVSS - afebrile, vital signs stable [Also AVSS]
3. ASA - acetylsalicylic acid (aspirin)
4. BD/BID - twice daily
5. BIBA - brought in by ambulance
6. BLS - basic life support
7. BP - blood pressure
8. BUN - blood urea nitrogen
9. C - Celsius; centigrade
10. Ca - calcium
11. CBC - complete blood count
12. Cl - chloride
13. cm - centimeter(s)
14. CNS - central nervous system
15. CO2 - carbon dioxide
16. COPD - chronic obstructive pulmonary (lung) disease
17. CPR - cardiopulmonary resuscitation
18. CSF - cerebrospinal fluid
19. CVA - cerebrovascular accident (stroke)
20. DM - diabetes mellitus
21. D/W - dextrose (a form of sugar) in water
22. ECG/EKG - electrocardiogram
23. EEG - electroencephalogram
24. EGD - esophagogastroduodenoscopy
25. ENT - ear, nose, and throat
26. ERCP - endoscopic retrograde cholangiopancreatography
27. F - Fahrenheit
28. FUO - fever of unknown origin
29. G, g - gram(s)
30. GFR - glomerular filtration rate
31. GI - gastrointestinal

32. GU - genitourinary
33. H,h,hr - hour(s)
34. Hb - hemoglobin
35. HCO3 - bicarbonate
36. HCT - hematocrit
37. HIPAA - Health Insurance Portability and Accountability Act
38. h/o - history of
39. HR - heart rate
40. hs - at bedtime
41. HTN - hypertension
42. I & D - incision and drainage
43. ICU - intensive care unit
44. IM - intramuscular
45. INR - international normalized ratio
46. IU - international unit
47. IV - intravenously
48. IVF - IV fluids
49. K - potassium
50. kcal - food calorie
51. kg - kilogram
52. L - liter
53. lb - pound
54. LDLc - low-density lipoprotein cholesterol
55. LLQ - left lower quadrant
56. LUQ - left upper quadrant
57. m - meter(m)
58. mEq - milliequivalent
59. mg - milligram
60. MI - myocardial infarction (heart attack)
61. Na - sodium
62. NaCl - sodium chloride
63. NPO - nothing by mouth
64. NSAID - nonsteroidal anti-inflammatory drug
65. NSR - normal sinus rhythm
66. n/v - nausea and vomiting
67. O2 - oxygen
68. OTC - over the counter

69. oz - ounce
70. P - pulse
71. PET - positron emission tomography
72. pH - hydrogen ion concentration
73. PO - orally
74. PR - per rectum
75. PRN - as needed
76. PT - prothrombin time
77. PTT - partial thromboplastin time
78. q - every
79. qid - 4 times daily
80. R - respiratory rate
81. RBC - red blood cells
82. RUQ - right upper quadrant
83. RLQ - right lower quadrant
84. SaO2 - arterial oxygen saturation
85. sc - subcutaneously
86. soln - solution
87. T - temperature
88. tid - 3 times daily
89. UA - urinalysis
90. URI - upper respiratory infection
91. WBC - white blood cells
92. wt - weight

Appendix 3

Glossary of Common Medical Terms

Below you will find definitions for various common medical terms you may hear your doctor use. Words in a term that are unfamiliar have an accompanying pronunciation key. The definitions are not exhaustive but give a good foundation for understanding common terms.

A
abscess [AB-sess] - a localized collection of pus
acute renal failure [REE-nal] - an abrupt decline in kidney function
adenoma [ad-e-NO-ma] - a noncancerous growth
akinesis [a-kin-EE-sis] - weak or absent movement, such as would occur in a portion of the heart after a massive heart attack
alkaline phosphatase [AL-ka-line FOS-fa-tase] - an enzyme that, when elevated, typically signifies liver or bone abnormalities
ALT - an enzyme that is a marker of liver injury or disease
alveoli [al-VEE-oe-lie] - tiny air sacs in the lungs used for gas exchange
amyloid [AM-i-loid] - an abnormal protein that can compromise the function of the organs it invades
anemia [a-KNEE-me-a] - a low concentration of red blood cells
aneurysm [AN-your-is-em] - a protrusion of a portion of the wall of an artery, veins or the heart
angina [AN-ji-na] - chest pain due to inadequate blood flow to the heart typically seen in patients with coronary artery disease
angiography [ann-gee-AWE-gra-fee] - a procedure that allows visualization of arteries
angioplasty [ANN-gee-oe-plas-tee] a procedure in which a tiny balloon is inserted in an artery and then inflated to lessen the extent of the artery's blockage

aortic insufficiency/regurgitation [A-or-tick] - leakiness of the aortic valve. The aortic valve is between the left ventricle and the aorta.
aortic stenosis [A-or-tick stin-O-sis] - narrowing of the aortic valve
arrhythmia [a-RITH-me-a] - an abnormal heart rhythm
arterial blood gases (ABGs) [ar-TEAR-ee-al] - a test of the gas content of the blood
arterial insufficiency [ar-TEAR-ee-al] - insufficient blood flow to an artery, usually due to atherosclerosis (hardening of the arteries)
arthrocentesis [ar-throw-cen-TEE-sis] - a test in which fluid is removed from a joint for evaluation
arthroscope [AR-throw-scope] - an instrument used to visualize the inside of a joint
arthroscopy [ar-THRAW-scope-ee] - a procedure used to examine the inside of a joint without open surgery
ascites [a-SITE-eez] - an excessive accumulation of fluid in the abdominal cavity
aspiration [as-per-A-shun] - 1: the act of inhaling; 2: withdrawing fluid from a joint or body cavity
AST - an enzyme that is a marker of liver injury or disease
asystole [ae-SIS-toe-lee] - when the heart stops beating, a form of cardiac arrest
atelectasis [at-el-ECK-us-is] - collapse of a portion of the lung
atherosclerosis [ath-er-oe-skler-O-sis] - hardening of the arteries due to deposition of cholesterol and other materials within the artery wall
atrial fibrillation [A-tree-al fi-bril-LAY-shun] - an abnormal heart rhythm that originates in the atria
atrial flutter [A-tree-al] - an abnormal heart rhythm that originates in the atria
atrial septal defect [A-tree-al SEP-tul] - a defect in the septum that separates the two atria
atrophy [A-tro-fee] - wasting away of a tissue or cell
AV block - a block in the electrical conduction system between the atria and ventricles
AV malformation - abnormal connections between arteries and veins

AV node - the part of the heart's electrical conduction system located at the junction of the atria and ventricles

B
bacteremia [bak-ter-EE-me-a] - the presence of bacteria in the bloodstream
bandemia [ban-DEE-me-a] - the presence of excessive bands in the bloodstream
bands - an immature population of a specific class of white blood cells
benign (BEE-nine) - noncancerous
bicarbonate [buy-CAR-bon-ate] - an indicator of the acid-base balance of the blood
bradycardia [bray-dee-CARD-ee-a] - a slow heart rate below 60 beats per minute
bronchodilator [bron-koe-DIE-late-or] - medication used to relieve spasm of tubes in the lungs thru which air travels; typically used in patients with asthma, COPD, and other lung diseases
bronchoscopy [bron-KAW-scope-ee] - a test done to visualize the lower airways
bronchospasm [BRON-koe-spaz-em] - spasm of a bronchus or airway
bronchus [BRON-kus] - a tube in the lung thru which air flows; the plural form is bronchi
bruit [BREW-ee] - an abnormal sound heard with a stethoscope that signifies blockage of a blood vessel
BUN (blood urea nitrogen) [your-EE-a] - an indicator of how well the kidneys are functioning
bundle branch block - a block in the branches of the electrical conduction system of the heart

C
CAD (coronary artery disease) - blockage of the arteries that supply the heart with blood
calcification [cal-si-fi-KAY-shun] - deposition of calcium in tissue

calculi [CAL-que-lie] - stones; plural of calculus; renal calculi are kidney stones
carcinoma [car-sin-O-ma] - a class of cancer
cardiac - pertaining to the heart
cardiac arrest [CAR-dee-ak] - when the heart stops beating
cardiac catheterization [CAR-dee-ak kath-e-ter-i-ZAY-shun] - a procedure that allows visualization of the arteries that supply the heart (coronary arteries) and evaluation of other important components of the heart
cardiomyopathy [car-dee-oe-my-OP-a-thee] - disease of the heart muscle
carotid [car-AWE-tid] - the two carotid arteries are the main arteries that supply blood to the brain
catheter [KATH-e-ter] - medical tube that can serve a variety of functions; a urinary catheter drains urine from the bladder
central nervous system - the brain and spinal cord
cerebral hemorrhage [sir-EE-bral] - bleeding into the brain tissue, such as with a certain type of stroke
cerebrospinal fluid [sir-ee-brow-SPINE-al] - the fluid that bathes the brain and spinal cord
cerebrovascular accident (CVA) [sir-ee-brow-VAS-que-lar] - a stroke
chloride - an important chemical in the blood
chronic obstructive pulmonary disease (COPD) - a term that generally refers to emphysema and/or chronic bronchitis
cirrhosis [sir-O-sis] - irreversible scarring of the liver, such as can occur with chronic alcohol abuse
claudication [claw-di-KAY-shun] - pain in the legs due to decreased blood flow/atherosclerosis
congestive heart failure - a common, treatable heart condition that leads to congestion of certain tissues with fluid
consolidation - solidification of tissue, such as in the lungs during pneumonia
coronary arteries - the arteries that supply the heart with blood

coronary artery disease [core-on-AIR-ee] - disease of the arteries that supply the heart with blood; the major cause of heart attacks

creatinine [kree-AT-in-een] - a test that indicates how well the kidneys are functioning

cyst [SIST] - a fluid-filled sac

cystitis [sis-TIGHT-is] - inflammation of the bladder usually due to infection

cytology studies [sigh-TOL-oe-gee] - microscopic examination of cells that can detect cancer

D

deep venous thrombosis (DVT) [VEE-nus throm-BOE-sis] - a blood clot in a vein that lies deep in the body, such as in a thigh or the pelvis

degenerative arthritis - routine 'wear and tear" arthritis, also known as osteoarthritis

demyelinating diseases [dee-MY-el-in-ate-ing] - diseases in which the coating of some nerve cells, called myelin, is disrupted. The most well-known example of a demyelinating disease is multiple sclerosis.

diastole [die-AS-toe-lee] - the portion of the cardiac cycle when the heart is relaxing

diastolic [die-a-STOL-ik] - pertaining to diastole; the diastolic blood pressure is the bottom number of a blood pressure reading

dyspnea [DISP-nee-a] - shortness of breath

dysrhythmia [dis-RITH-me-a] - an abnormal heart rhythm, also called an arrhythmia

E

echocardiogram (ECHO) [ek-oe-CARD-ee-oe-gram] - an ultrasound study of the heart

effusion [ee-FEW-shun] - an excessive accumulation of fluid

electrocardiogram [ee-lec-troe-CARD-ee-oe-gram]- commonly called an EKG; a test is which shows the electrical activity of the heart

electrophysiologic studies [ee-leck-troe-fizz-ee-oe-LOJ-ic] - electrical studies done to evaluate patients with known or suspected abnormal heart rhythms

embolism [EM-bow-lis-em] - abrupt blockage of an artery by a blood clot or other material that dislodged from elsewhere; a pulmonary embolism is a blood clot in a lung

empyema [em-pie-E-ma] - a collection of pus in the space between the lungs and chest wall, called the pleural space

endocarditis [en-dough-car-DITE-is] - inflammation of the heart valves, usually due to infection

endometrium [en-dough-ME-tree-um] - the internal lining of the uterus

endoscope [EN-doe-scope] - an instrument used to visualize internal body structures

erythrocytes [e-RITH-row-sites] - red blood cells

esophageal varices [ee-SOF-a-gee-al var-i-SEES] - enlarged blood vessels in the wall of the esophagus

esophagogastroduodenoscopy (EGD) [ee-SOF-a-go-gas-troe-do-od-en-AWE-scope-ee] - an endoscopic procedure that allows a doctor to view the upper part of the gastrointestinal tract

esophagram [ee-SOF-a-gram] - another name for the barium swallow test; it allows for examination of the esophagus

exudate [EX-you-date] - material that has escaped from blood vessels due to inflammation or other abnormalities

F

fatty liver - infiltration of the liver by fat cells

fibroadenoma [fir-broe-ad-en-O-ma] - a noncancerous growth in the breast

fibroids [FIE-broids] - noncancerous masses in the uterus that can cause excessive menstrual bleeding or pain, or interfere with a pregnancy

fibrosis [fie-BROE-sis] - scarring

fistula [FIST-you-la] - an abnormal passage, often between two organs but sometimes between an organ and the surface of the body

forced expiratory volume in one second (FEVI) - an important indicator of airway obstruction seen in lung disease
forced vital capacity (FVC) - the amount of air you can force from your lungs after taking your deepest breath

G
gastric ulcer [GAS-trick UL-cer] - a stomach ulcer
gastric varices [GAS-trick VER-i-sees] - enlarged blood vessels in the stomach, often due to cirrhosis
gastritis [gas-TRY-tis] - inflammation of the lining of the stomach
gastroesophageal reflux disease (GERD) [gas-troe-ee SOF-a-gee-al] - a common condition characterized by refluxing of stomach acid upward into the esophagus, frequently causing heartburn
glomeruli [glow-MER-you-lie] - collection of small blood vessels that are used by the kidneys to filter waste; the kidney's functional units
glomerulonephritis [glow-mer-you-low-nef-RIGHT-is] - inflammation of the glomeruli
glucose [GLUE-cose] - blood sugar
glycohemoglobin [gly-co-HEME-a-globe-in] (also called A1c or Hemoglobin A1C) - a test that evaluates how well diabetes has been controlled over the past two or three months
goiter [GOY-ter] - an enlarged thyroid gland
granulocytes [GRAN-you-low-sites] - an important class of white blood cells
granuloma [gran-you-LOW-ma] - a noncancerous collection of cells
guaiac test [GWIE – ak] (also called hemoccult test) – a test for occult blood, such as blood in the stool

H
HDL cholesterol (high-density lipoprotein) - a negative risk factor for coronary artery disease; high levels give some degree protection against heart disease
hematocrit [he-MAT-oe-crit] - a measure of the volume of red blood cells in the bloodstream

hematoma [he-ma-TOE-ma] - a collection of blood, usually clotted, due to disruption of a local blood vessel (may look like a big bruise)
hematuria [he-ma-TURE-ee-a] - blood in the urine
heme - an important component of red blood cells
heme-negative stools - the test did not detect any occult blood in the stool
heme-positive stools - the test did detect occult blood in the stool
hemoccult [HE-mow-cult] test (also called guaiac) - a common test to detect inconspicuous (or occult) heme, a component of red blood cells; most frequently done to test stool
hemoglobin [HE-mow-globe-in] - the oxygen-carrying component of red blood cells
hemoglobin A$_{1c}$ [HE-mow-globe-in) - a test to assess how well diabetes has been controlled over the past two to three months; abbreviated HbA$_{1c}$
hemorrhage - bleed
hepatic (he-PAT-ic] - pertaining to the liver
hydronephrosis [high-droe-ne-FROW-sis] - distention of a part of the kidney due to obstruction, such as from a kidney stone
hypercalcemia [high-per-cal-SEEM-ee-a] - a high blood calcium concentration
hypercholesterolemia [high-per-koe-les-ter-ol-EE-me-a] - high blood cholesterol level
hyperinflation [high-per-in-FLAY-shun] - over inflation of the lungs
hyperkalemia [high-per-kay-LEEM-ee-a] - a high blood potassium concentration
hypernatremia [high-per-nay-TREE-me-a] - a high blood sodium concentration
hypoxemia [high-pox-EE-me-a] - deficient oxygen content of the blood

I
infarction [in-FARK-shun] - death of tissue; a myocardial infarction is a heart attack; a cerebral infarction is a stroke
inverted T waves - upside-down T waves seen on an EKG. They often indicate compromised blood flow to the heart.

ischemia [is-KEY-me-a] - a condition in which body tissue lacks adequate blood flow; chest pain due to ischemia is common with blocked arteries in the heart

J K L

junctional rhythm - an abnormal heart rhythm that originates at the junction between the atria and ventricles in the heart

ketones (KEY-tones) - a product of metabolism that can be found in excessive amounts in the blood or the urine under certain circumstances, such as in poorly controlled diabetes

lateral – position relative to the outer side of the body; the shoulder is lateral to the neck

LDL cholesterol (low-density lipoprotein) - a powerful risk factor that, when high, increases the chances of developing coronary artery disease (CAD)

leads - an EKG consists of 12 leads, or angles, for recording the electrical activity of the heart

left atrial enlargement [A-tree-all] - enlargement of the left atrium of the heart

left bundle branch block - a block in the bundle of electrical fibers on the left side of the heart's conduction system

left ventricle [VEN-trick-ul] - the largest chamber of the heart

left ventricular hypertrophy (LVH) [ven-TRICK-you-lar high-PER-troe-fee] - enlargement of the muscular wall of the left ventricle

leukocyte esterase [LUKE-oe-site ES-ter-ase] - a screening test for white blood cells in the urine, a potential sign of a urinary tract infection

leukocytes [LUKE-oe-sites] - another name for white blood cells. There are different classes of leukocytes, which include:
- **Polymorphonuclear leukocytes (PMNs)** [pol-ee-mor-foe-NEW-clee-ar]
- **Lymphocytes** [LIMP-foe-sites]
- **Monocytes** [MON-oe-sites]
- **Basophils** [BASE-oe-fils]
- **Eosinophils** [ee-oe-SIN-oe-fils]

leukocytosis [luke-oe-site-O-sis] - an increased number of circulating white blood cells

lipid [LIP-id] - a fatty substance found in the bloodstream and in cell walls, among other places

lipoprotein [lie-poe-PRO-teen] - water-soluble molecules capable of transporting water-insoluble lipids (fats) in the bloodstream, such as LDL (low-density lipoprotein) cholesterol and HDL (high-density lipoprotein) cholesterol

M

medial – position relative to the center or middle; the breastbone is medial to the arm

metastasis [mu-TA-stas-is] - a cancerous mass that has spread from its primary location

mitral insufficiency/regurgitation [MY-tral] - leakiness of the mitral valve of the heart. The mitral valve is between the left atrium and left ventricle.

mitral stenosis [MY-tral stin-O-sis] - narrowing of the mitral valve of the heart

mitral valve prolapse (MY-tral valve PRO-lapse) - an abnormal upward motion of a portion of the mitral valve during contraction of the heart

multiorgan system failure - the failure of several organs, such as occurs in septic shock

myocardial [my-oe-CARD-ee-al] - pertaining to heart muscle

myocardial infarction [my-oe-CARD-ee-al in-FARK-shun] - a heart attack

N

necrosis [ne-CROW-sis] - death of tissue; necrotic tissue is dead tissue

neoplasm [NEE-oe-plaz-em] - an abnormal growth that may be benign or malignant

nephrolithiasis [ne-froe-lith-I-as-is] - kidney stones

neuropathy [nur-OP-a-thee] - a disturbance of a nerve or nerves

nitrites [NIGH-trites] - a substance that, when found in the urine, suggests a urinary tract infection

nontoxic goiter [GOY-ter] - an enlarged, but not overactive, thyroid gland

O

organomegaly [or-gan-oe-MEG-a-lee] - an enlarged organ; often used to describe conditions of the liver or spleen

osteoarthritis [os-tee-oe-ar-THRITE-is] - routine "wear and tear," or degenerative, arthritis

P

paracentesis [pair-a-cent-E-sis] - withdrawal of fluid from the abdominal cavity

paroxysmal supraventricular tachycardia (PSVT) [pair-ox-IS-mal sue-pra-ven-TRICK-you-lar tack-ee-CARD-ee-a] - a very rapid heart rate that originates above the ventricles

patella [pa-TELL-a] - knee bone

peak inspiratory flow rate - the rate of air flow when you take your deepest breath

perfusion [per-FEW-shun] - refers to blood flow

pericardial effusion [pair-ee-CARD-ee-al ee-FEW-shun] - increased fluid in the sac surrounding the heart

plaque [PLAK] - when pertaining to the arteries, plaques refer to a buildup of cholesterol-rich material that blocks the inside of the artery

platelets [PLATE-e-lets] - important blood clotting particles

pleurae [PLUR-a] - two membranes that line the outer surface of the lungs and the inner surface of the chest wall

pleural effusion [PLUR-al ee-FEW-shun] - an abnormal accumulation of (pleural) fluid in the space between the pleural membranes

pleural space [PLUR-al] - the space between the two pleural membranes, one on the outer surface of the lungs and the other on the inner surface of the chest wall

pneumothorax [new-moe-THOR-ax] - a collapsed lung

proteinuria [pro-teen-YOUR-ee-a] - protein in the urine
pulmonary [PULL-mon-air-ee] - a term that refers to the lungs
pulmonary angiography [PULL-mon-air-ee an-gee-AWE-graf-ee] - a test done to visualize the blood vessels of the lungs
pulmonary edema [PULL-mon-air-ee e-DEEM-a] - fluid accumulation within the lung tissue
pulmonary embolism [PULL-mon-air-ee EM-bow-lis-em] - a blood clot in the lungs that originated elsewhere, such as in the thigh
pulmonary hypertension [PULL-mon-air-ee] - elevated pressure in the blood vessels of the lungs
pulmonary insufficiency/regurgitation [PULL-mon-air-ee] - leakiness of the valve that controls blood flowing from the right ventricle to the lungs, the pulmonary valve.
P waves - waves on an EKG that indicate electrical - excitation of the atria
pyelonephritis [pie-el-oe-nef-RIGHT-is] - a kidney infection

Q
QRS complex- represents the electrical activity seen on an EKG that leads to contraction of the ventricles
Q wave - EKG evidence of a scar in the heart tissue typically signifying a prior heart attack

R
renal [REE-nal] -pertaining to the kidneys
renal calculi [REE-nal CAL-que-lie] - kidney stones
right atrial enlargement [A-tree-al] - enlargement of the right atrium of the heart
right bundle branch block - a block in the bundle of electrical fibers on the right side of the conduction system of the heart
right ventricle [VEN-trick-ul] - one of the heart's four chambers
right ventricular hypertrophy [ven-TRICK-you-lar high-PER-troe-fee] - enlargement of the muscular wall of the right ventricle of the heart

S

sepsis [SEP-sis] - the body's extreme response to a serious infection, usually including fever, a fast heart rate, and rapid breathing

septic arthritis - infection of the joint

septic shock - advanced sepsis which results in a low blood pressure and often failure of multiple organs, or multiorgan system failure

septum [SEP-tum] - a wall of tissue that divides chambers, such as heart chambers

sigmoid [sig-MOID] - a portion of the end of the colon

sinus arrhythmia [a-RITH-me-a] - a slightly abnormal, although usually clinically insignificant, heart rhythm

sinus node - the heart's natural pacemaker

sinus rhythm - the normal rhythm of the heart

spirometry [spy-ROM-e-tree] - the most basic part of the pulmonary function tests

ST depression - depression of the ST segment on the EKG, usually representing compromised blood flow

ST elevation - elevation of the ST segment on the EKG, often suggestive of an acute heart attack

stenosis [stin-O-sis] - narrowing

strain - when discussing EKG results, a variation of the ST segment of the EKG often seen in patients with left ventricular hypertrophy

stricture [STRIK-chur] - a decrease in the caliber of a passageway

ST segment - an important segment of the cardiac cycle seen on an EKG. When elevated or depressed the heart may be deprived of oxygen,

sublingual [sub-LEEN-gwal] - under the tongue

synovial fluid [sin-oe-VEE-al] - lubricating fluid that decreases friction in joints

systole [SIS-toe-lee] - the portion of the cardiac cycle when the heart is contracting; the systolic blood pressure is the top number of the blood pressure

T

tachycardia [tack-ee-CARD-ee-a] - a fast heart rate, greater than 100 beats per minute

thoracentesis [thor-a-cent-EE-sis] - a procedure in which a needle is inserted into the thorax, usually to withdraw fluid for analysis

thrombophlebitis [throm-boe-flee-BITE-is] - inflammation in a vein due to a blood clot

thrombosis [throm-BOE-sis] - a blood clot that can occur in an artery or vein

tidal volume - the amount of air you inhale and exhale during a normal respiratory cycle

total/HDL ratio - the ratio of total cholesterol to HDL cholesterol. This ratio gives information about the overall risk of coronary artery disease.

transient ischemic attack (TIA) [is-KEY-mic] - a "mini-stroke;" symptoms are short-lived and there is no lasting damage to the brain

transudate [TRANS-you-date] - fluid containing a low concentration of protein and cell components

tricuspid insufficiency/regurgitation [try-CUS-pid] - leakiness of the tricuspid valve of the heart. The tricuspid valve is between the right atrium and right ventricle.

tricuspid stenosis [try-CUS-pid stin-O-sis] - narrowing of the tricuspid valve of the heart

triglyceride [try-GLIS-er-ide] - a fatty substance found in the blood linked to heart disease

T waves - relaxation of the ventricles seen on an EKG

U

ureter [YOUR-e-ter] – tubes which drain the urine from the kidneys to the bladder

ureteral obstruction [your-EE-ter-al] - obstruction of the ureters

urinalysis [your-in-AL-is-is] - analysis of the urine

V W X Y Z

valvular heart disease [VAL-view-lar] - a generic term designating an abnormality of one or more of the four heart valves

valvular regurgitation/insufficiency [VAL-view-lar] - leakiness of a valve

valvular stenosis [VAL-view-lar stin-O-sis] - narrowing of a heart valve

varicosities [var-i-KOS-it-ees] - varicose veins

vegetation - mass on a heart valve seen with an infection of the heart valve

venipuncture [VEEN-i-punk-shur] - puncturing a vein to take a blood sample

ventricular aneurysm [ven-TRICK-you-lar AN-your-is-em] - a protrusion of the wall of the ventricle

ventricular fibrillation [ven-TRICK-you-lar fib-ri-LAY-shun] - a deadly heart rhythm; a form of cardiac arrest

ventricular mural thrombus [ven-TRICK-you-lar MURE-al THROM-bus] - a blood clot attached to the inside wall of the ventricle

ventricular septal defect [ven-TRICK-you-lar SEP-tal] - a defect in the septum that separates the two ventricles of the heart

ventricular tachycardia [ven-TRICK-you-lar tack-ee-CARD-ee-a] - a potentially serious heart rhythm that can deteriorate into a cardiac arrest in some cases

vital capacity - the amount of air that you can blow out after taking your deepest breath

V/Q mismatch - a mismatch between the areas of the lung that exchange air and the areas that should receive blood, which suggests the possibility of a pulmonary embolus

V/Q scan ventilation (V)/perfusion (Q) scan - test done to test for a blood clot in the lungs, a pulmonary embolism

X-ray – a special picture of a body part

Patient Empowerment Books
By Dr. Ann M. Hester

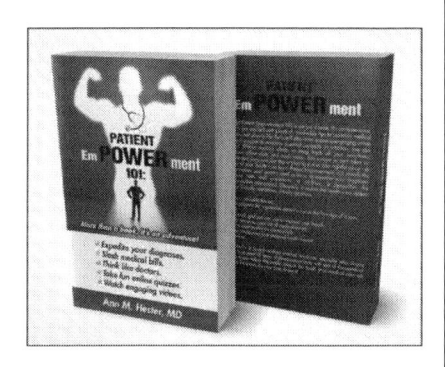

Available in paperback and Kindle eBook formats.

Available in paperback format.

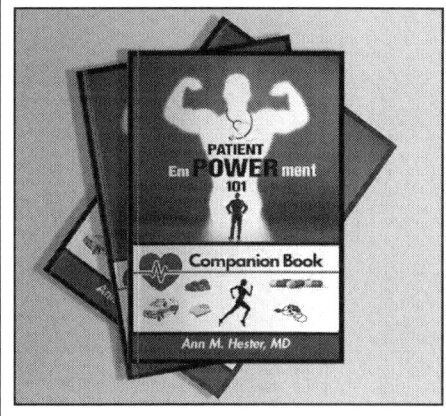

Fillable charts, questionnaires, and notes sections bring the book to life!

Webpages

https://www.patientempowerment101.com/my-records

https://www.patientempowerment101.com/symptoms

https://www.patientempowerment101.com/quizzes

https://www.patientempowerment101.com/videos

Made in the USA
Columbia, SC
16 March 2023